# CORRIGENDA

## 2010 Report
## Tuberculosis Control in the Western Pacific Region

ISBN 978 92 9061 522 4

(NLM Classification: WF 200)

**Page xii:** Summary Table, Table 1. Main TB indicators 2008
Incidence and CDR: all forms <u>number</u> (not rate)
ss+ <u>number</u> (not rate)

**Page 96:** Table 61. Estimated prevalence and prevalent cases of MDR-TB in selected countries and areas in the Region, 2008, should read as follows:

| Country | Source of estimates | % MDR among new TB cases (95% CI) | % MDR among previosly treated TB cases (95% CI) | Number of MDR-TB among incident new and relapse TB cases (95% CI) | Number of incident acquired MDR-TB cases (95% CI) | Number among incident total TB cases (95% CI) |
|---|---|---|---|---|---|---|
| Australia | model | 2.2 (0.0–10.7) | 10.8 (0.0–34.5) | 19 (9–33) | 1 (0–2) | 21 (9–32) |
| Brunei Darussalam | model | 2.2 (0.0–10.7) | 10.8 (0.0–34.5) | 11 (0–29) | 1 (0–3) | 12 (0–26) |
| Cambodia | DRS | 0.0 (0.0–0.6) | 3.1 (1.1–8.8) | 2000 (112–4900) | 200 (0–580) | 2200 (0–4600) |
| China | DRS | 5.7 (5.0–6.6) | 25.6 (22.6–28.3) | 84 000 (65 000–106 000) | 15 000 (12 000–20 000) | 100 000 (79000–120 000) |
| Cook Islands | model | 1.9 (0.0–7.5) | 13.8 (0.0–36.2) | 0 (0–0) | 0 (0–0) | 0 (0–0) |
| Fiji | model | 1.9 (0.0–7.5) | 13.8 (0.0–36.2) | 5 (0–12) | 1 (0–2) | 5 (0–11) |
| Japan | DRS | 0.7 (0.5–1.1) | 9.8 (7.3–13.1) | 220 (130–340) | 64 (43–87) | 290 (180–390) |
| Kiribati | model | 1.9 (0.0–7.5) | 13.8 (0.0–36.2) | 10 (1–24) | 1 (0–3) | 11 (0–22) |
| Lao People's Democratic Republic | model | 1.9 (0.0–7.5) | 13.8 (0.0–36.2) | 270 (13–650) | 8 (0–23) | 280 (0–590) |
| Malaysia | DRS | 0.1 (0.0–0.6) | 0.0 (0.0–19.4) | 31 (1–120) | 74 (0–210) | 104 (0–220) |
| Marshall Islands | model | 1.9 (0.0–7.5) | 13.8 (0.0–36.2) | 4 (0–9) | 0 (0–1) | 4 (0–8) |
| Federated States of Micronesia | model | 1.9 (0.0–7.5) | 13.8 (0.0–36.2) | 3 (0–7) | 0 (0–0) | 3 (0–6) |
| Mongolia | DRS | 1.0 (0.4–2.5) | 13.8 (0.0–36.2) | 63 (17–140) | 43 (0–120) | 110 (21–190) |
| Nauru | model | 1.9 (0.0–7.5) | 13.8 (0.0–36.2) | 0 (0–0) | 0 (0–0) | 0 (0–0) |
| New Zealand | DRS | 0.0 (0.0–1.6) | 0.0 (0.0–39.0) | 15 (1–37) | 1 (0–2) | 15 (0–33) |
| Niue | model | 1.9 (0.0–7.5) | 13.8 (0.0–36.2) | - | - | - |
| Palau | model | 1.9 (0.0–7.5) | 13.8 (0.0–36.2) | 0 (0–1) | 0 (0–0) | 0 (0–1) |
| Papua New Guinea | model | 1.9 (0.0–7.5) | 13.8 (0.0–36.2) | 530 (9–1300) | 73 (0–210) | 600 (0–1200) |
| Philippines | DRS | 4.0 (3.0–5.5) | 20.9 (14.8–28.7) | 11 000 (7300–15 000) | 2000 (1100–3000) | 13 000 (8900–17 000) |
| Republic of Korea | DRS | 2.7 (2.1–3.4) | 14.0 (10.4–18.6) | 1400 (1000–1700) | 490 (300–700) | 1900 (1400–2300) |
| Samoa | model | 1.9 (0.0–7.5) | 13.8 (0.0–36.2) | 1 (0–2) | 0 (0–0) | 1 (0–2) |
| Singapore | DRS | 0.1 (0.0–0.6) | 2.9 (1.0–8.2) | 2 (0–9) | 1 (0–3) | 4 (0–8) |
| Solomon Islands | model | 1.9 (0.0–7.5) | 13.8 (0.0–36.2) | 18 (1–43) | 3 (0–7) | 20 (0–42) |
| Tonga | model | 1.9 (0.0–7.5) | 13.8 (0.0–36.2) | 1 (0–2) | 0 (0–0) | 1 (0–2) |
| Tuvalu | model | 1.9 (0.0–7.5) | 13.8 (0.0–36.2) | 0 (0–1) | 0 (0–1) | 1 (0–1) |
| Vanuatu | DRS | 0.0 (0.0–11.7) | 13.8 (0.0–36.2) | 5 (0–12) | 0 (0–1) | 5 (0–11) |
| Viet Nam | DRS | 2.7 (2.0–3.6) | 19.3 (14.5–25.2) | 5600 (3700–8100) | 280 (180–420) | 5900 (3800–8100) |

## 2010 Report

# Tuberculosis Control

## in the Western Pacific Region

**Prepared by**

Masaki Ota, Research Institute of Tuberculosis, Tokyo, was the lead author of this report. The following WHO staff from the regional and country offices contributed to the report: Catharina van Weezenbeek, Pieter van Maaren, Daniel Sagebiel, Katsunori Osuga, Nobuyuki Nishikiori, Catherine Lijinsky, Rajendra Yadav, Cornelia Hennig, Fabio Scano, Liu Yuhong, Nguyen Nhat Linh, Jacques Sebert, Yamuna Mundade, Woo-Jin Lew and Giampaolo Mezzabotta.

Correspondence: stoptb@wpro.who.int

**Acknowledgements**

We would like to thank the national TB Control Programme (NTP) managers and statisticians from all countries and areas of the Western Pacific Region for providing data for this publication and to the Stop TB team in the TB Monitoring and Evaluation unit at WHO Headquarters responsible for the Global TB Report. Also, we would like to express our gratitude to the US Agency for International Development (USAID) and Japan Voluntary Contribution (JVC), which kindly provided funds to support this report.

WHO Library Cataloguing in Publication Data

**Tuberculosis control in the Western Pacific Region: 2010 Report**

**1. Tuberculosis – epidemiology. 2. Tuberculosis – prevention and control. 3. Tuberculosis – drug therapy. 4. Directly observed therapy – utilization. 5. Tuberculosis, Multidrug-resistant. 6. Western Pacific.**

ISBN **978 92 9061 522 4** (NLM Classification: **WF 200**)



Layout and design by Alexander Pascual, www.alexdesigns.ph

# Contents

# List of figures

# List of tables

# List of abbreviations

| | |
|---|---|
| **ART** | antiretroviral therapy |
| **CI** | confidence interval |
| **CPT** | cotrimoxazole preventive therapy |
| **DOTS** | directly observed treatment, short-course |
| **DRS** | drug resistance surveillance |
| **DST** | drug susceptibility testing |
| **EQA** | external quality assessment |
| **GLC** | Green Light Committee |
| **HIV** | human immunodeficiency virus |
| **IDU** | injecting drug users |
| **IPT** | isoniazid preventive therapy |
| **MDR-TB** | multidrug-resistant tuberculosis |
| **NAP** | National AIDS Control Programme |
| **NTP** | National Tuberculosis Control Programme |
| **PICs** | Pacific island countries and areas |
| **PMDT** | Programmatic management of drug resistant TB |
| **pop.** | population |
| **ss+ or ss-** | sputum smear-positive or sputum smear-negative |
| **SRLN** | supranational laboratory network |
| **TB** | tuberculosis |
| **WHO** | World Health Organization |

# Executive summary

The 2010 report on tuberculosis (TB) control in the WHO Western Pacific Region presents data on disease burden, case notification in 2008 and treatment outcomes for patients registered in 2007. The report also includes information on drug resistant-TB, TB-HIV coinfection, laboratory services, profiles of the seven countries with a high burden of TB in the Region—Cambodia, China, Lao People's Democratic Republic, Mongolia, Papua New Guinea, the Philippines, and Viet Nam—and a summary of the epidemiological indicators and treatment outcomes in the Pacific island countries and areas. The report seeks to provide an update on the current epidemiological situation of TB and to show progress in TB control in the Region.

The report highlights the following:

### TB burden

There were an estimated 2.1 million prevalent TB cases (120 per 100 000 population) in the Region in 2008, of which 1.9 million were incident cases (109 per 100 000 population), including 0.9 million new smear-positive cases (53 per 100 000 population). The estimated number of incident cases accounted for 21% of the global burden of TB. In absolute numbers, China, the Philippines, Viet Nam and Cambodia ranked first to fourth, respectively. These four countries accountec for 93% of the total estimated incident cases in the Region. Cambodia had the highest incidence rate (490 per 100 000 population). Death from TB occurred in about 0.3 million cases (15 per 100 000 population). The mortality rate was the highest in Cambodia (79 per 100 000 population).

### Case notification and trends

The Region accounted for about 1.4 million cases of all forms of TB notified in 2008 (76 per 100 000 population), corresponding to 24% of the total cases notified globally. There were about 0.7 million new sputum smear-positive cases (37 per 100 000 population) notified, corresponding to 25% of the global smear-positive cases notified. The largest number of smear-positive cases were notified from China (463 000), followed by the Philippines (85 000) and Viet Nam (53 000). Since 2005, the notification rates for all forms of TB and new sputum smear-positive TB have remained stable in the Region.

### Progress towards 2010 regional goal

The 2010 Regional goal was to halve the TB prevalence and mortality rates from those of the year 2000. Between 2000 and 2008, the TB prevalence rate is estimated to have declined by 46% at a rate of -7.5% per year and the mortality rate by 42% at a rate of -6.6% per year. At the current rates of decline, the prevalence will drop from 224 to 103 per 100 000 population by 2010 and the mortality from 26 to 13 per 100 000 population.

### Treatment outcomes

Of the 0.7 million new pulmonary smear-positive cases registered for treatment in 2007, the overall treatment success rate was 92% in the Region. Treatment success rates were above the 85% target in six of seven countries with a high burden of TB: Cambodia, China, Lao People's Democratic Republic, Mongolia, the Philippines and Viet Nam. Only Papua New Guinea did not reach the target, with 39% treatment success (for most cases, no treatment outcome available).

### Multidrug-resistant TB

The estimated number of incident MDR-TB cases among all forms of TB (new and relapse) in the Region was about 120 000 (6.2%), of which cases from China, the Philippines and Viet Nam accounted for 97% of the overall total MDR-TB cases. Prevalence of MDR-TB reported between 2000 and 2008 varied from country to country and also by treatment history of the patient. In five countries with a high burden of TB for which data from surveys were available—Cambodia, China, Mongolia, the Philippines and Viet Nam—MDR-TB prevalence in new cases ranged from 0% in Cambodia to 5.7% in China and in retreatment cases from 3.1% in Cambodia to 27.5% in Mongolia (preliminary data for 2008).

### TB-HIV coinfection

Among the countries and areas that reported the TB-HIV data, about 150 000 patients of 1.4 million notified cases of all forms of TB were tested for HIV in 2008. The proportion of TB cases tested for HIV increased from 9.3% in 2007 to 11% in 2008. Of 150 000 tested, about 11 000 (6.9%) were found to be HIV-positive. In the Region, the overall estimated prevalence of HIV in new TB cases was 2.3%.

### Laboratory services

In 2008, there were 6981 TB laboratories that performed acid-fast bacilli (AFB) smear microscopy in the seven countries with a high burden of TB in the Region, of which 6460 (93%) participated in external quality assessment (EQA) programmes. In five of the seven countries with a high burden of TB—Cambodia, China, Lao People's Democratic Republic, Mongolia and Viet Nam—over 95% of sputum smear microscopy centres participated in EQA activities.

In the seven countries with a high burden of TB in the Region, there were a total of 666 laboratories capable for TB culture in 2008. In six of the seven high burden countries—Cambodia, China, Mongolia, Papua New Guinea, the Philippines and Viet Nam—some 666 AFB culture facilities have been established, of which 117 are capable of performing DST for the first-line anti-TB drugs. The Lao People's Democratic Republic just started culture and DST after completion of the National Reference Laboratory in August 2009. However, the number of laboratories in the Region capable of performing culture and DST is insufficient, given the threat of MDR-TB and TB-HIV coinfection.

# Summary Table

**Table 1.** Main TB indicators 2008

| | | Notified cases (DOTS + non-DOTS) | | | | | Incidence and CDR | | | Cure/Success | |
|---|---|---|---|---|---|---|---|---|---|---|---|
| | | New + relapse | | New pulmonary | | | Est. incidence | | CDR | 2007 ss+ cohort | |
| | | (WHO total) | | ss+ | | | | | | | |
| | Population thousands | number | rate | number | rate | ss-/unk. number | all forms rate | ss+ rate | All new % | Cured % | Success % |
| American Samoa | 67 | 3 | 5 | | | 3 | 2 | 1 | 140 | | |
| Australia | 21 074 | 1213 | 6 | 299 | 1 | 409 | 1400 | 340 | 87 | 7 | 85 |
| Brunei Darussalam | 392 | 223 | 57 | 132 | 34 | 28 | 260 | 150 | 87 | 63 | 76 |
| Cambodia | 14 562 | 38 927 | 267 | 19 860 | 136 | 7847 | 71 000 | 35 000 | 55 | 91 | 94 |
| China | 1 337 411 | 975 821 | 73 | 462 596 | 35 | 431 115 | 1 300 000 | 640 000 | 75 | 93 | 94 |
| Cook Islands | 20 | 2 | 10 | 2 | 10 | | 4 | 2 | 50 | 0 | 100 |
| Fiji | 844 | 106 | 13 | 78 | 9 | 5 | 170 | 82 | 64 | 81 | 81 |
| French Polynesia | 266 | 50 | 19 | 20 | 8 | 18 | 58 | 23 | 87 | 85 | 85 |
| Guam | 176 | 89 | 51 | 31 | 18 | 50 | 100 | 36 | 87 | 89 | 89 |
| Hong Kong (China) | 6982 | 5544 | 79 | 1459 | 21 | 2981 | 6400 | 1700 | 87 | 59 | 66 |
| Japan | 127 293 | 24 181 | 19 | 8995 | 7 | 8856 | 28 000 | 10 000 | 87 | 17 | 46 |
| Kiribati | 110 | 335 | 304 | 147 | 133 | 71 | 350 | 170 | 97 | 79 | 93 |
| Lao People's Democratic Republic | 6–205 | 4–048 | 65 | 3–079 | 50 | 519 | 9300 | 4600 | 44 | 91 | 92 |
| Macao (China) | 526 | 359 | 68 | 139 | 26 | 150 | 410 | 160 | 87 | 49 | 91 |
| Malaysia | 27 014 | 17 144 | 63 | 10 441 | 39 | 3 814 | 28 000 | 14 000 | 62 | 67 | 72 |
| Marshall Islands | 61 | 125 | 206 | 28 | 46 | 62 | 130 | 63 | 98 | 93 | 96 |
| Federated States of Micronesia | 97 | 164 | 169 | 38 | 39 | 89 | 100 | 51 | 160 | 25 | 65 |
| Mongolia | 2641 | 4490 | 170 | 1838 | 70 | 640 | 5400 | 2700 | 83 | 85 | 89 |
| Nauru | 10 | 5 | 50 | 2 | 20 | 2 | 1 | 1 | 420 | 0 | 100 |
| New Caledonia | 246 | 44 | 18 | 9 | 4 | 22 | 51 | 10 | 87 | 69 | 77 |
| New Zealand | 4230 | 292 | 7 | 101 | 2 | 91 | 340 | 120 | 87 | 0 | 86 |
| Niue | 1 | 0 | 0 | 0 | 0 | 0 | | | | | |
| Commonwealth of the Northern Mariana Islands | 85 | 28 | 33 | 13 | 15 | 12 | 32 | 15 | 87 | 0 | 92 |
| Palau | 21 | | | | | | 13 | 6 | 0 | | |
| Papua New Guinea | 6577 | 13 984 | 213 | 2323 | 35 | 5340 | 16 000 | 8100 | 85 | 33 | 39 |
| Philippines | 90 348 | 139 603 | 155 | 85 025 | 94 | 49 916 | 260 000 | 130 000 | 54 | 79 | 89 |
| Republic of Korea | 48 152 | 36 847 | 77 | 11 048 | 23 | 17 292 | 42 000 | 13 000 | 87 | 81 | 82 |
| Samoa | 179 | 12 | 7 | 6 | 3 | 5 | 33 | 16 | 37 | 85 | 92 |
| Singapore | 4615 | 1549 | 34 | 526 | 11 | 672 | 1800 | 600 | 87 | 62 | 81 |
| Solomon Islands | 511 | 387 | 76 | 140 | 27 | 136 | 620 | 310 | 63 | 75 | 92 |
| Tokelau | 1 | | 0 | | 0 | | | | | | |
| Tonga | 104 | 13 | 13 | 11 | 11 | | 24 | 12 | 53 | 93 | 93 |
| Tuvalu | 10 | 17 | 170 | 9 | 90 | 5 | 16 | 8 | 110 | 56 | 75 |
| Vanuatu | 234 | 103 | 44 | 45 | 19 | 19 | 170 | 86 | 59 | 81 | 93 |
| Viet Nam | 87 096 | 97 772 | 112 | 53 484 | 61 | 19 056 | 170 000 | 86 000 | 56 | 89 | 92 |
| Wallis and Futuna | 15 | | | | | | 1 | | 0 | | |
| **Western Pacific Region** | **1 788 175** | **1 363 480** | **76** | **661 924** | **37** | **549 225** | **1 942 185** | **947 362** | **70** | **89** | **92** |

ss+ = sputum smear-positive; ss-= sputum smear-negative; unk. = sputum smear result unknown; est. = estimated; CDR = case detection rate; re-treat. = retreatment; rcvd. = received

* 2008 value / 2000 value, expressed as a percentage. The 2010 goal is 50%.

| HIV-TB | MDR-TB | | Prevalence | | | Mortality | | | |
|---|---|---|---|---|---|---|---|---|---|
| Est. prevalence in adult incident TB cases (%) | Retreat-ment cases received DST number | MDR in re-treatment cases number | 2000 All forms rate | 2008 All forms rate | All forms change* | 2000 All forms rate | 2008 All forms rate | All forms change* | |
| 100 | | 0 | 2 | 1 | 69% | 0 | 0 | | American Samoa |
| 2.3 | 33 | 4 | 4 | 5 | 115% | 0 | 0 | 233% | Australia |
| 0 | | 0 | 98 | 43 | 44% | 5 | 4 | 89% | Brunei Darussalam |
| 15 | 91 | 28 | 1000 | 680 | 68% | 110 | 79 | 72% | Cambodia |
| 1.7 | | 0 | 210 | 88 | 42% | 25 | 12 | 48% | China |
| | | 0 | 3 | 32 | 1143% | 0 | 4 | 816% | Cook Islands |
| 3.3 | | 0 | 30 | 25 | 83% | 4 | 3 | 80% | Fiji |
| | 2 | 0 | 8 | 6 | 71% | 2 | 1 | 72% | French Polynesia |
| 3.3 | | 0 | 19 | 61 | 321% | 3 | 4 | 160% | Guam |
| 0.51 | 390 | 14 | 58 | 58 | 100% | 7 | 6 | 88% | Hong Kong (China) |
| 0.49 | | 0 | 23 | 12 | 52% | 2 | 1 | 64% | Japan |
| 0 | | 0 | 490 | 110 | 22% | 64 | 25 | 39% | Kiribati |
| 2 | | 0 | 360 | 260 | 72% | 42 | 32 | 76% | Lao People's Democratic Republic |
| 0.25 | 25 | 2 | 68 | 49 | 72% | 7 | 5 | 69% | Macao (China) |
| 12 | | 0 | 140 | 120 | 86% | 17 | 15 | 88% | Malaysia |
| 0 | | 0 | 510 | 59 | 12% | 60 | 14 | 23% | Marshall Islands |
| 0 | 3 | 0 | 130 | 34 | 26% | 17 | 7 | 39% | Federated States of Micronesia |
| 0.15 | 334 | 114 | 230 | 140 | 61% | 30 | 21 | 70% | Mongolia |
| | | 0 | 50 | 10 | 20% | 7 | 1 | 12% | Nauru |
| | 4 | 0 | 51 | 10 | 20% | 4 | 1 | 37% | New Caledonia |
| 1 | 11 | 0 | 3 | 5 | 173% | 0 | 1 | 165% | New Zealand |
| | | 0 | 4 | | | 0 | 0 | | Niue |
| 0 | | 0 | 110 | 11 | 10% | 8 | 2 | 27% | Commonwealth of the Northern Mariana Islands |
| | | 0 | 23 | 110 | 478% | 4 | 14 | 378% | Palau |
| 3.8 | | 0 | 130 | 130 | 100% | 21 | 21 | 100% | Papua New Guinea |
| 0.26 | 1305 | 729 | 780 | 550 | 71% | 66 | 52 | 79% | Philippines |
| 0.53 | | 0 | 16 | 50 | 313% | 9 | 6 | 62% | Republic of Korea |
| | | 0 | 20 | 36 | 180% | 3 | 4 | 154% | Samoa |
| 2.5 | 103 | 3 | 32 | 27 | 84% | 3 | 3 | 78% | Singapore |
| | | 0 | 360 | 150 | 42% | 43 | 19 | 44% | Solomon Islands |
| | | 0 | | | ! | 0 | 0 | | Tokelau |
| 0 | | 0 | 29 | 22 | 76% | 4 | 3 | 79% | Tonga |
| 0 | | 0 | 190 | 44 | 23% | 26 | 11 | 42% | Tuvalu |
| | | 0 | 79 | 88 | 111% | 11 | 11 | 100% | Vanuatu |
| 3.8 | | 0 | 290 | 280 | 97% | 36 | 34 | 94% | Viet Nam |
| | | 0 | 140 | 2 | 1% | 16 | 0 | 2% | Wallis and Futuna |
| **2.3** | **2301** | **894** | **224** | **120** | **54%** | **26** | **15** | **58%** | **Western Pacific Region** |

# 1 Introduction

This is the annual report on tuberculosis (TB) control published by WHO's Regional Office for the Western Pacific. Geographically and economically, the Western Pacific Region—which covers East Asia and the Pacific—has a great diversity of natural and human resources, economic dynamism, technological expertise and agricultural productivity. The Region has a total population of 1788 million, representing about 27% of the world's population. In 2008, the Region accounted for 21% of the estimated global TB incidence and 19% of the prevalence, respectively.

Each year 36 countries and areas[1] in the Region report data to WHO using a standardized collection form for reporting surveillance data. Using data on disease burden and case notifications in 2008 and treatment outcomes of patients registered for treatment in 2007, this report presents an assessment of TB epidemiology, burden, estimation and progress towards the Regional goal to halve the prevalence and mortality rates of 2000 by 2010[2] and to achieve at least 85% successful treatment for new smear-positive cases and a case detection rate of 70%. This report includes data on drug resistance, TB-HIV surveillance, laboratory services and TB prevalence surveys conducted between 2000 and 2008 within the Region.

In addition, the report provides country- and area-specific data, which include epidemiologic indicators and detailed estimations of prevalence and mortality towards the 2010 goal for seven countries and areas with a high burden of TB. The epidemiological indicators and treatment outcomes of TB for the Pacific island countries are also summarized. There are nine annexes.

The first four describe methods for estimating prevalence and mortality for past, current and future years and the burden of multidrug-resistant TB[3] (MDR-TB) and provide definitions. In Annex 5, the names and contact information of the partners in countries with a high burden of TB in the Region are listed. Annex 6 provides explanatory notes for the tables listed in Annex 7. Subnational data on all forms of TB are in Annex 8. Notified prevalence of resistance to antiTB drugs and estimated numbers of MDR-TB cases that had occurred in 2008 are in Annex 9.

The case detection rate (CDR) has been a much-used indicator of national progress in TB control since the mid-1990s. This report only presents estimates of the CDR for all new cases using the methodology of "Global Tuberculosis Control–a short update to the 2009 report" (WHO/HTM/TB/2009.426). Concerning the most recent development of moving away from estimates of the case detection rate for sputum smear-positive pulmonary TB please refer to chapter 4.3 and Box 6 of "Global Tuberculosis Control 2010" (WHO/HTM/TB/2010.7).

1 See Table 1 for countries and areas in the Region.

2 The regional goal differs from the Millennium Development Goals.

3 Isolates that are resistant to at least isoniazid and rifampicin.

# 2 Epidemiology

## 2.1 Estimated burden

**Figure 1.** Estimated incident cases of all forms of TB by WHO Region, 2008

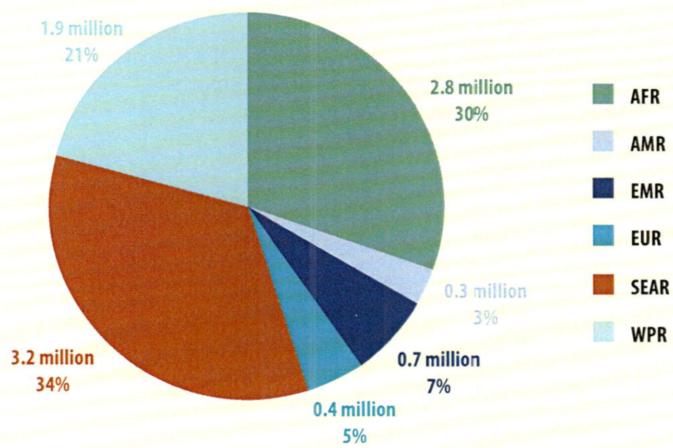


**AFR** = African Region; **AMR** = American Region; **EMR** = East Mediterranean Region;
**EUR** = European Region; **SEAR** = Southeast Asia Region; **WPR** = Western Pacific Region

In 2008, there were an estimated 2.1 million prevalent TB cases (120 per 100 000 population) in the Region. Over 1.9 million were incident cases (109 per 100 000 population), including 0.9 million new smear-positive cases (53 per 100 000 population). The estimated number of incident cases accounts for 21% of the global burden of TB (Figure 1). Figure 2 shows the estimated incidence rates of TB by country and area.

The incidence rate was the highest in Cambodia (490 per 100 000 population). Cases from Cambodia, China, the Philippines and Viet Nam together accounted for 93% of all incidence cases in the Region. Prevalence of all forms of TB declined at an estimated rate of 7.5% annually since 2000 (Table 2). Death from TB was estimated to occur in about 260 000 cases in 2008 (15 per 100 000 population). The mortality rate was highest in Cambodia (79 per 100 000 population) and lowest in American Samoa, Australia, Niue and Tokelau (0 per 100 000 population). Deaths from TB in Cambodia, China, the Philippines and Viet Nam accounted for 95% of all TB mortality in the Region. The regional TB mortality rate declined at an estimated rate of 6.6% annually since 2000 (Table 2).

**Table 2.** Estimated prevalence (all forms of TB) and TB mortality per 100 000 population in the Region, 2008

| | Year | | Overall decline 2000–2008 | Annual decline 2000–2008 |
|---|---|---|---|---|
| | 2000 | 2008 | | |
| Estimated Prevalence | **224 [150–332]** | **120 [61 -196]** | 46% | 7.5% |
| Estimated Mortality | **26 [10 -49]** | **15 [6 -30]** | 42% | 6.6% |

*The ranges around the best estimates in this table show the highest and lowest estimates.

**Figure 2.** Estimated incidence rates (left) and prevalence rates (right) of all forms of TB by country and territory, 2008

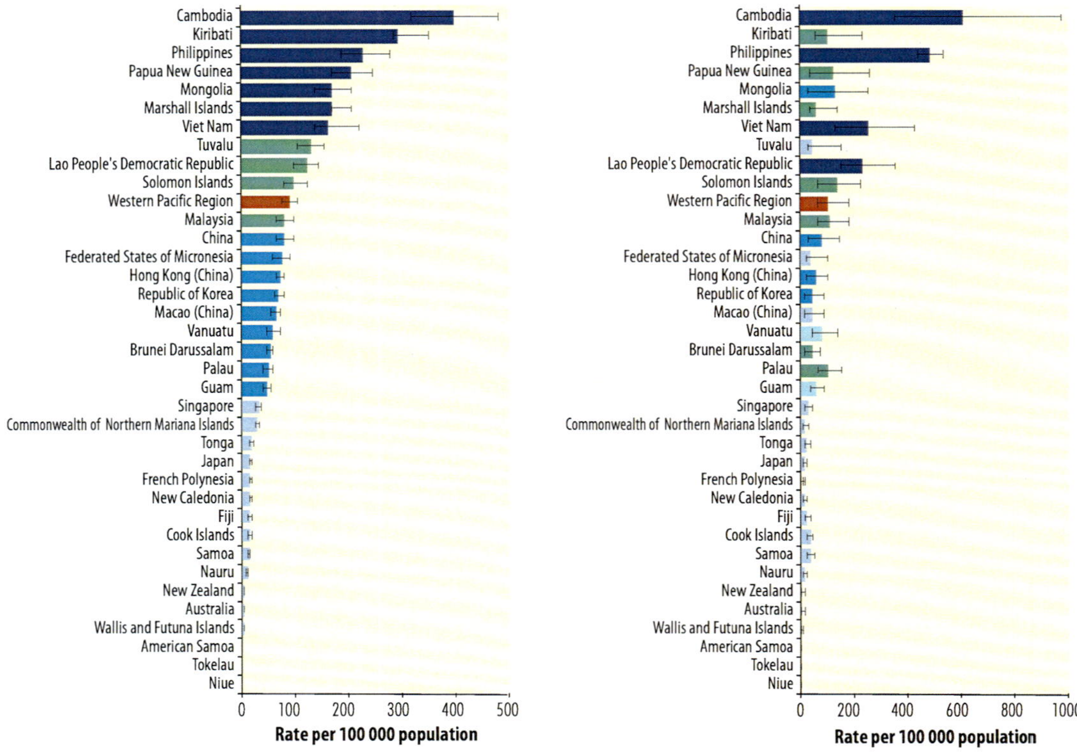


WPR = Western Pacific Region

*The bars show the boundaries within which the actual rates lie, based on the best available information .

**Figure 3.** Distribution of estimated incident cases (all forms) by country and area in the Region, 2008 (n = 1 942 185 )

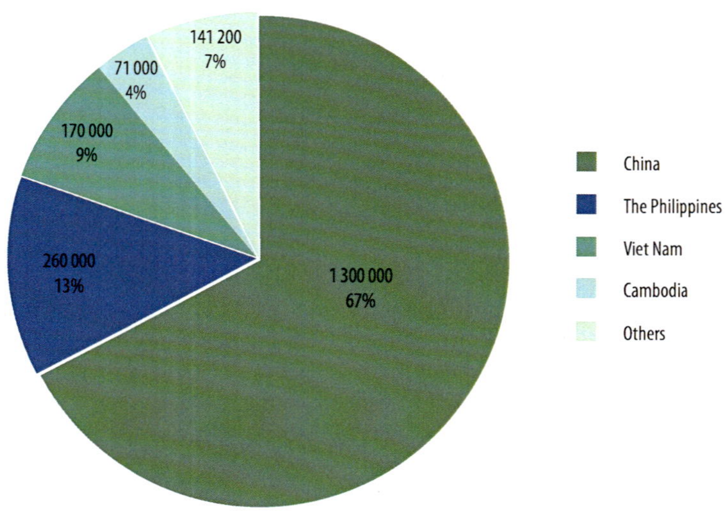


## 2.2 Trend of prevalence and TB mortality rates in countries with a high burden of TB

Regionally, prevalence and mortality had declined at rates of 7.5% per year and 6.6% per year, respectively, since 2000. At the current rate of decline, in 2010 the prevalence would be 103 and the mortality 13 per 100 000 population (see estimation method in Annex 1) (Table 3). Thus, according to the latest WHO estimates, the regional goal of halving prevalence and mortality by 2010 relative to 2000 levels is likely to be achieved whereas it would most likely not have been met with the previous method of estimation. However, the latest WHO estimates have large confidence intervals and thus should be interpreted with care.

**Table 3.** Estimated TB prevalence and mortality in 2010 by country and area with a high burden of TB in the Region and Regional 2010 goals

| Country and area | Prevalence rate | | | | Mortality rate | | | |
|---|---|---|---|---|---|---|---|---|
| | Overall change 2000–2008 (%) | Annual rate of decline[a] (%) | Estimate in 2010* | 2010 goal† | Overall change 2000–2008 (%) | Annual rate of decline[a] (%) | Estimate in 2010* | 2010 goal† |
| Cambodia | 32 | 4.7 | 617 | 500 | 28 | 4.1 | 73 | 55 |
| China | 58 | 10.3 | 71 | 105 | 52 | 8.8 | 10 | 13 |
| Lao People's Democratic Republic | 28 | 4.0 | 240 | 180 | 24 | 3.3 | 30 | 21 |
| Mongolia | 39 | 6.0 | 124 | 115 | 30 | 4.4 | 19 | 15 |
| Papua New Guinea | 0 | 0.0 | 130 | 65 | 0 | 0.0 | 21 | 11 |
| Philippines | 29 | 4.3 | 504 | 390 | 21 | 2.9 | 49 | 33 |
| Viet Nam | 3 | 0.4 | 278 | 145 | 6 | 0.7 | 34 | 18 |
| **Western Pacific Region** | **46** | **7.5** | **103** | **112** | **42** | **6.6** | **13** | **13** |

[a] Average from 2000 through 2008
* Per 100 000 population, assuming current rate of change
† Assuming current annual rate of change

## 2.3 Case notification and trends

About 1.4 million cases of all forms of TB were notified in 2008 (76 per 100 000 population), corresponding to 24% of the total cases notified globally. There were 0.7 million new smear-positive cases notified in 2008 (37 per 100 000 population), corresponding to 25% of the total smear-positive cases notified globally. The largest number of smear-positive cases was reported from China (463 000), followed by the Philippines (85 000) and Viet Nam (53 000). Together with Cambodia, cases from these four countries accounted for 94% of all new smear-positive cases notified in the Region. Two countries with a high burden of TB in the Region, Cambodia and Papua New Guinea, had case notification rates of ≥200 per 100 000 population. Figure 4 shows case notification rates for all forms of TB in countries and areas in the Western Pacific Region and neighbouring countries and areas in 2008.

**Figure 4.** Case notification rates (all forms of TB) per 100 000 population in countries and areas in the Western Pacific Region and neighbouring countries and areas, 2008

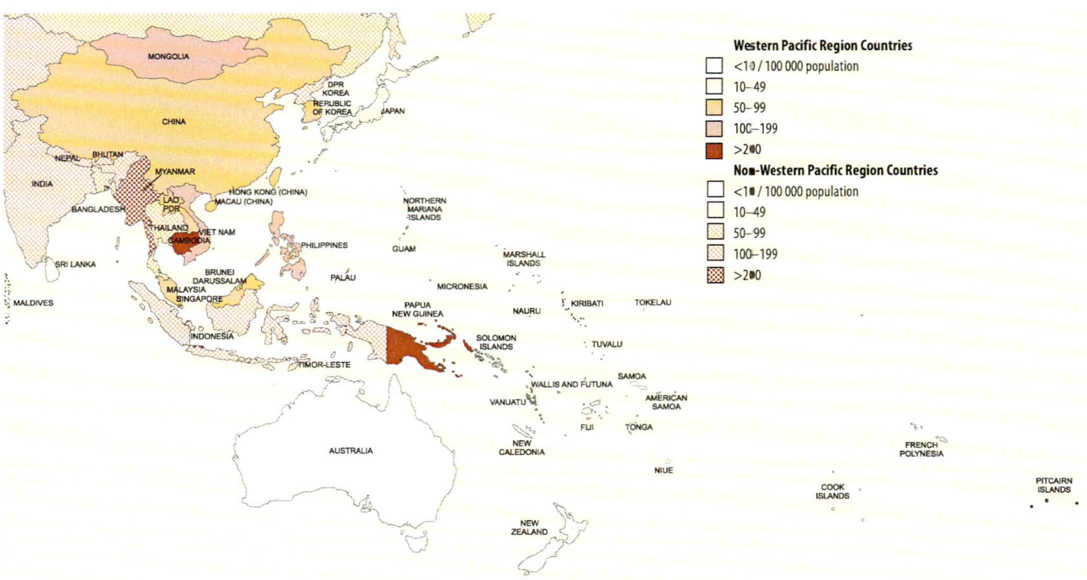


The boundaries shown and the designations used on this map do not imply the expression of any opinion whatsoever on the part of WHO concerning the legal status of any country, territory, city or area or of its authorities, or concerning the delimitation of its frontiers or boundaries. White lines on maps represent approximate border lines for which there may not yet be full agreement. 

Between 2002 and 2005, the case notification rates in the Region had increased from 47 to 73 per 100 000 population in all forms of TB (trend +15% per year) and from 22 to 38 per 100 000 population in new smear-positive TB cases (trend +19% per year). After 2005, the case notification rates in new smear-positive cases and in all forms of TB have stabilized (Figure 5).

**Figure 5.** Case notification rates (all forms of TB and smear-positive cases) in the Region, 2000–2008

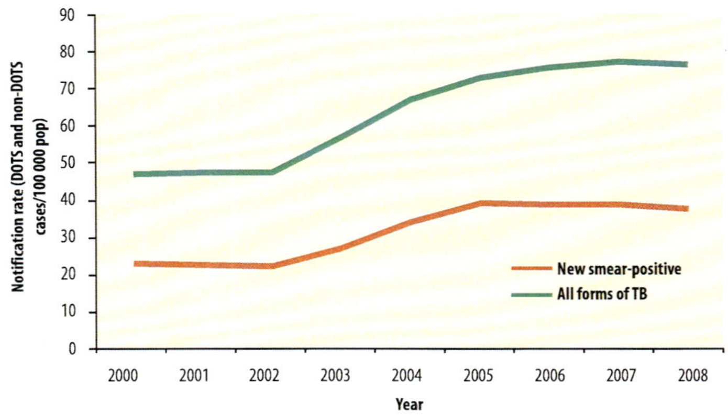


Figure 6 shows age- and sex-specific case notification rates (new smear-positive) for the seven countries with a high burden of TB in the Region. In general, TB disproportionately affected males except for Papua New Guinea, where both males and females are almost equally affected. For every female smear-positive TB case older than 15 years old, 1.1 (Papua New Guinea) to 3.0 (Viet Nam) male smear-positive TB cases were notified. Older age groups are more likely to develop TB in these seven countries, except for Mongolia, Papua New Guinea and the Philippines, where TB more frequently occurred in those younger than 65 years old.

**Figure 6.** Smear-positive notification rates by age and sex in the Region and in seven countries with a high-burden of TB, 2008

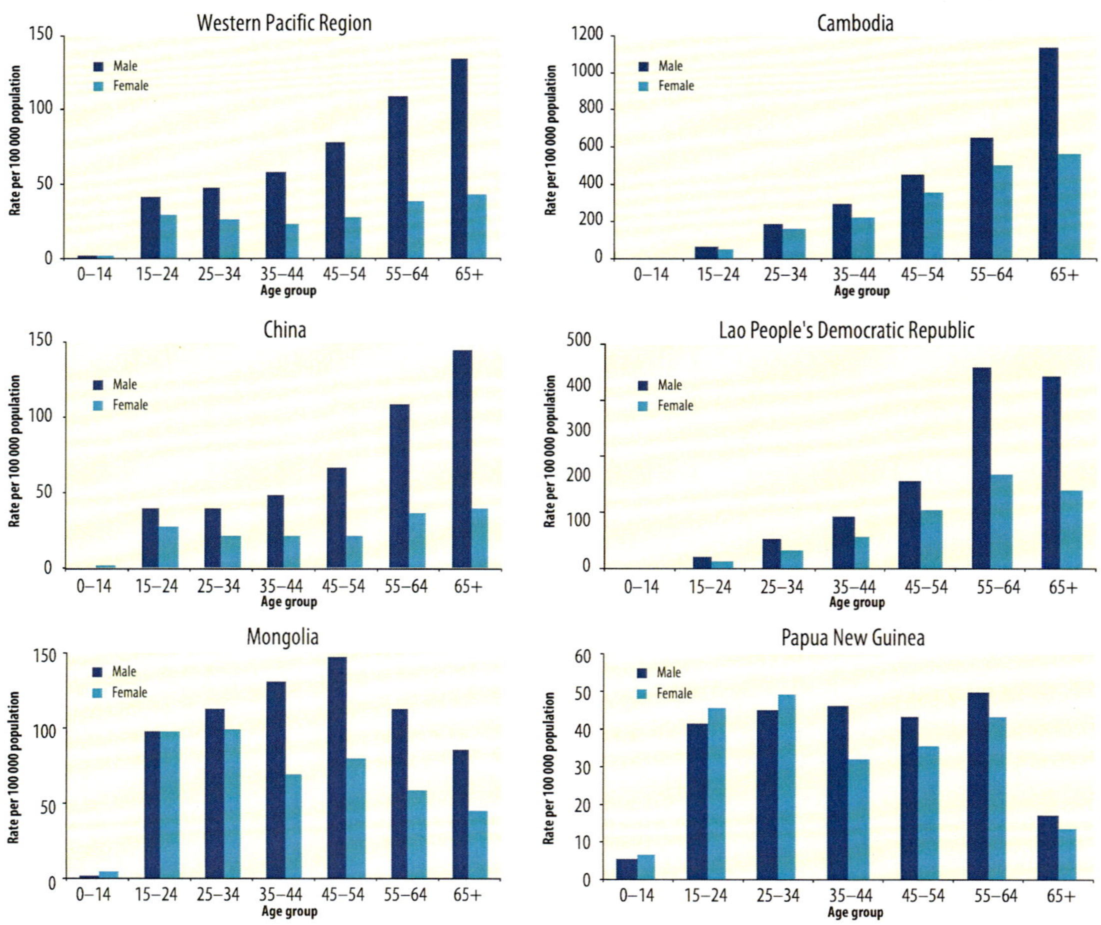

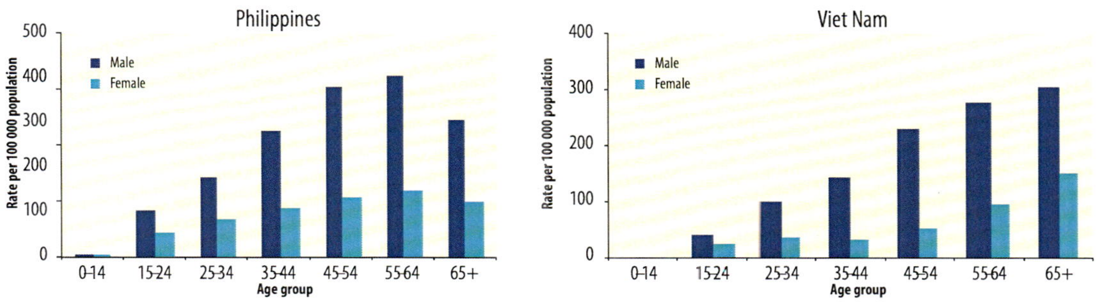


**Figure 7.** The distribution of sex ratio (male to female) of notified smear-positive cases by age group in Cambodia and Viet Nam, 2008

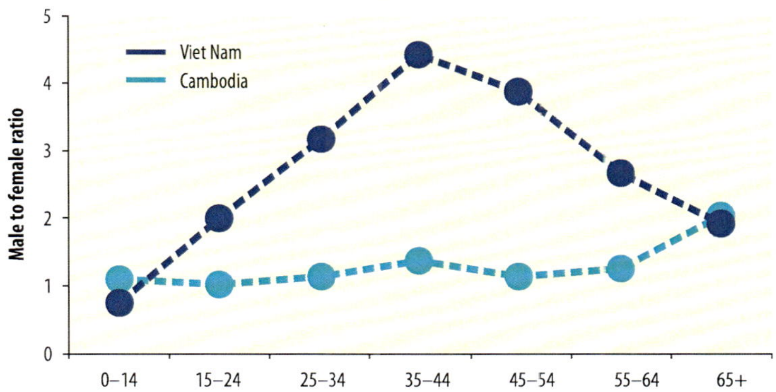


As in previous years, the distribution of sex ratio of notified smear-positive cases by age group in Cambodia and Viet Nam show very different patterns (Figure 7). The sex ratio is consistently close to one through all age groups except the group 65 years old or older in Cambodia, while the ratio is more than two among those 25 years old or older in Viet Nam.

Trends in age group- and sex-specific notification rates reflect underlying epidemiological processes of TB infection. Stable or increasing notification rates in a certain age group, particularly in young adults, are an indicator of continuing transmission in the population. With low or no continuing transmission in a population, new cases of TB largely will occur among those already infected (i.e. the older age groups) and the notification rates in all age groups will decline. In a country which experiences demographic changes, trends of overall notification rates may not seem to change while specific trends in certain age group- and sex-specific notification rates may reveal further findings.

Figure 8 shows notification rates of new smear-positive cases of overall and of age- and sex-specific groups in Viet Nam between 2000 and 2008. The overall notification rate for smear-positive cases did not show a decrease between 2000 and 2004. However, the analysis of the notification rates stratified by age group and sex showed that there was a decrease in males in the 35-year-old or older age groups and in females in 25-year-old or older age groups during that period. The rising notification rates in young adults (15–34-year- old age group in males and 15–24-year-old age group in females) offset the overall decline expected from TB control activities in the country. After 2004, the overall notification rate for new smear-positives started to decrease, facilitated by the reverse of the trend in young male adults (15–34 years old), particularly after 2006. However, the notification rates in young adult females has remained stable (25–34-year-old age group) or rising (15–24-year-old age group), partly caused by the rapid increase in HIV-TB coinfected patients in young adults.[4]

4 Meeting report: The fifth Technical Advisory Meeting to Stop TB in the Western Pacific Region, WHO/WPRO, 2006

**Figure 8.** Trends of notification rates of new smear-positive TB cases in overall (upper graph) and in specific age and sex groups (lower graphs), Viet Nam, 2000–2008

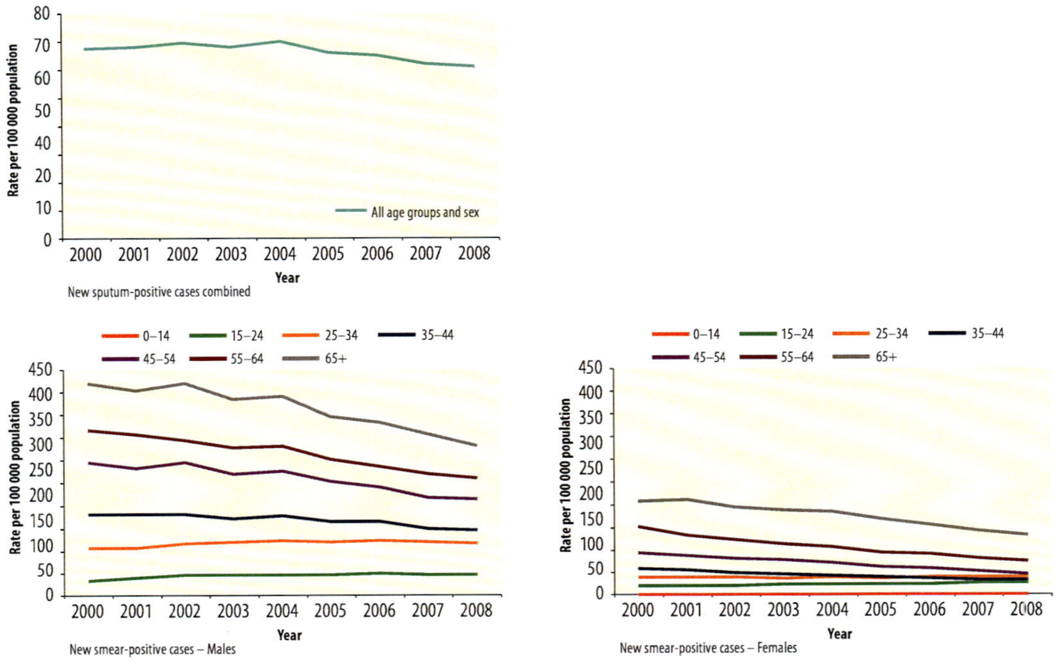


## 2.4 TB prevalence surveys

TB prevalence is one of the most important indicators to assess how well TB control has performed in a country. However, estimating prevalence of TB using TB notification data has some limitations due to TB surveillance limitations in general, particularly where access to health care facilities is limited (both geographically and financially), the quality of laboratory services is not assured or reporting from health care facilities (private and/or public) is incomplete. TB prevalence surveys allow direct measurement of the TB burden in a country or area in a specific time period.

The WHO Global Task Force on TB Impact Measurement has identified 21 priority countries recommended to conduct prevalence surveys between 2008 and 2015; four of those countries are in the Western Pacific Region: Cambodia, China, the Philippines and Viet Nam. The Philippines (2007) and Viet Nam (2006) have completed surveys, with subsequent surveys planned close to 2015. Cambodia and China will implement surveys in 2010 following previous surveys conducted in 2002 (Cambodia) and in 1990 and 2000 (China). In addition, a prevalence survey was to be conducted in the Lao People's Democratic Republic in 2010 for the first time. The results of previous surveys in the countries between 2000 and 2008 are summarized in Table 4.

**Table 4.** Summary of results of prevalence surveys conducted in the Region, 2000–2008

| Country | Year | No. of subjects participated | Prevalence rate (/100 000 pop.) | |
|---|---|---|---|---|
| | | | ss+ (95% C.I.) | bac+* (95% C.I.) |
| Cambodia | 2002 | 22 160 | 362 (284–461) | 1208 (997–1463) |
| China | 2000 | 365 097 | 122 (108–137) | 160 (143–177) |
| Philippines | 2007 | 22 867 | 200 (120–270) | 470 (360–580) |
| Viet Nam | 2006 | 93 251 | 136 (99–173) | 214 (168–261) |

No. = number; pop. = population; ss+ = sputum smear-positive; bac+ = bacteriologically positive; C.I. = confidence interval
*The definition of "bacteriologically positive TB" depends on surveys; either smear- and culture- positive or only culture-positive cases fall into the definition.

TB prevalence surveys also provide NTPs with additional useful information on smear- and culture-positive TB. Further, they allow for a comparison with routine surveillance data. Male-to-female ratios of notification and prevalence rates, as well as duration of illness, are shown in Table 5. Duration of illness of males in Cambodia (2.2) and Viet Nam (1.8, insignificant) is longer, while in the Philippines the duration of illness is shorter in males than in females (0.8, insignificant). Here, gender-specific differences in health-seeking behaviour, patients and/or diagnostic delay and biological factors may play a role.

**Table 5.** Male-to-female ratios of notification and prevalence rates and duration of illness

| Country | Year | Prevalence rate (/100 000 pop.) | | |
|---|---|---|---|---|
| | | notification rr (ss+) | prevalence rr (ss+) (95%C.I.) | duration of illness (ss+) (95%C.I.) |
| Cambodia | 2002 | 1.2 | 2.6 (1.4–3.8) | 2.2 (1.1–3.2) |
| Philippines | 2007 | 2.4 | 1.8 (0.80–2.8) | 0.77 (0.35–1.2) |
| Viet Nam | 2006 | 2.8 | 4.9 (2.3–7.5) | 1.8 (0.83–2.7) |

rr = rate ratio; ss+ = sputum smear-positive; C.I. = confidence interval

Male to female ratios of duration of illness was calculated from the equation shown below:

$$\text{Male to female ratio of duration of illness} = \frac{\dfrac{\text{prevalence rate (male)}}{\text{notification rate (male)}}}{\dfrac{\text{prevalence rate (female)}}{\text{notification rate (female)}}}$$

China not listed (data by sex not available)

## 2.5 Drug resistance

Between 2000 and 2008, 21 countries and areas in the Region have conducted at least one round of drug resistance surveillance (DRS) in collaboration with the Global Project on Antituberculosis Drug Resistance Surveillance established in 1994. TB strains resistant to any of the first-line anti-TB drugs were found in all settings surveyed in the Region except for Fiji and Solomon Islands (Table 6 and Annex 9). The prevalence of MDR-TB varied from country to country and by treatment history of the patient.

Among new TB cases in the Region, the MDR-TB prevalence ranged from 0% in Cambodia to 11.1% in the Commonwealth of the Northern Mariana Islands. In retreatment cases, it ranged from 2.9% in Singapore to 27.5% in Mongolia. In five countries with a high burden of TB for which surveyed data were available (Cambodia, China, Mongolia, the Philippines and Viet Nam), MDR-TB prevalence in new cases ranged from 0% in Cambodia to 5.7% in China and in retreatment cases from 3.1% in Cambodia to 27.5% in Mongolia (preliminary data for 2008).

**Table 6.** AntiTB drug resistance in recent surveys, by country and area, 2005–2008 (see Annex 9 for more detailed data)

| Country and area | Year | Case notification | | | | Retreatment cases | |
|---|---|---|---|---|---|---|---|
| | | No. of strains tested | INH resistance (%) | Any resistance (%) | MDR | No. of strains tested | MDR (%) |
| Australia* | 2008 | 887 | 8.7 | 10.8 | 2.4 | - | - |
| China | 2007 | 3037 | 16.0 | - | 5.7 | 892 | 25.6 |
| Fiji* | 2006 | 38 | 0.0 | 0.0 | 0.0 | - | - |
| Hong Kong (China) | 2008 | 2443 | 4.3 | 9.4 | 0.3 | 310 | 3.2 |
| Japan†* | 2007 | 1859 | 3.0 | 9.2 | 0.8 | - | - |
| Macao (China) | 2008 | 243 | 2.5 | 8.6 | 2.1 | 25 | 4.0 |
| Mongolia† | 2008 | 650 | - | 16.6 | 1.4 | 200 | 27.5 |
| New Caledonia* | 2005 | 5 | 20.0 | 20.0 | 0.0 | - | - |
| New Zealand† | 2007 | 211 | 4.7 | 9.0 | 0.0 | 14 | 14.3 |
| Commonwealth of the Northern Mariana Islands | 2006 | 18 | 22.2 | 16.7 | 11.1 | - | - |
| Republic of Korea | 2008 | 2581 | 9.6 | 11.8 | 3.1 | 731 | 12.3 |
| Singapore | 2008 | 919 | 2.3 | 6.3 | 0.1 | 103 | 2.9 |
| Vanuatu | 2006 | 29 | 3.4 | 3.4 | 0.0 | - | - |
| Viet Nam | 2006 | 1619 | 30.7 | 19.1 | 2.7 | 207 | 19.3 |

No. = number; INH = isoniazid; MDR-TB = multidrug-resistance tuberculosis

* Combined new and retreatment cases

† Preliminary results, some data were not yet available.

China conducted a nationwide DRS in 2007. While the details about the survey design have not been reported, the values for drug resistance are very close to those estimated in the past from subnational studies. It was shown that 5.7% of new cases and 25.6% of previously treated cases had MDR-TB. Notably, data from recent surveys in five of China's 31 provinces revealed alarming rates of MDR-TB in more than half of these provinces (Figure 9 and 10), with MDR-TB among new TB cases ranging between 2% and 10%, substantially higher than the global average. It was greater than 7% among new TB cases in three provinces—Henan, Heilongjiang and Inner Mongolia—that had implemented a successful DOTS programme for nearly 10 years, indicating that implementing DOTS alone may not be sufficient to control the MDR-TB epidemic in China.

**Figure 9.** Geographic distribution of MDR-TB among new cases by country and area in the Region and by province in China, 2000–2008*

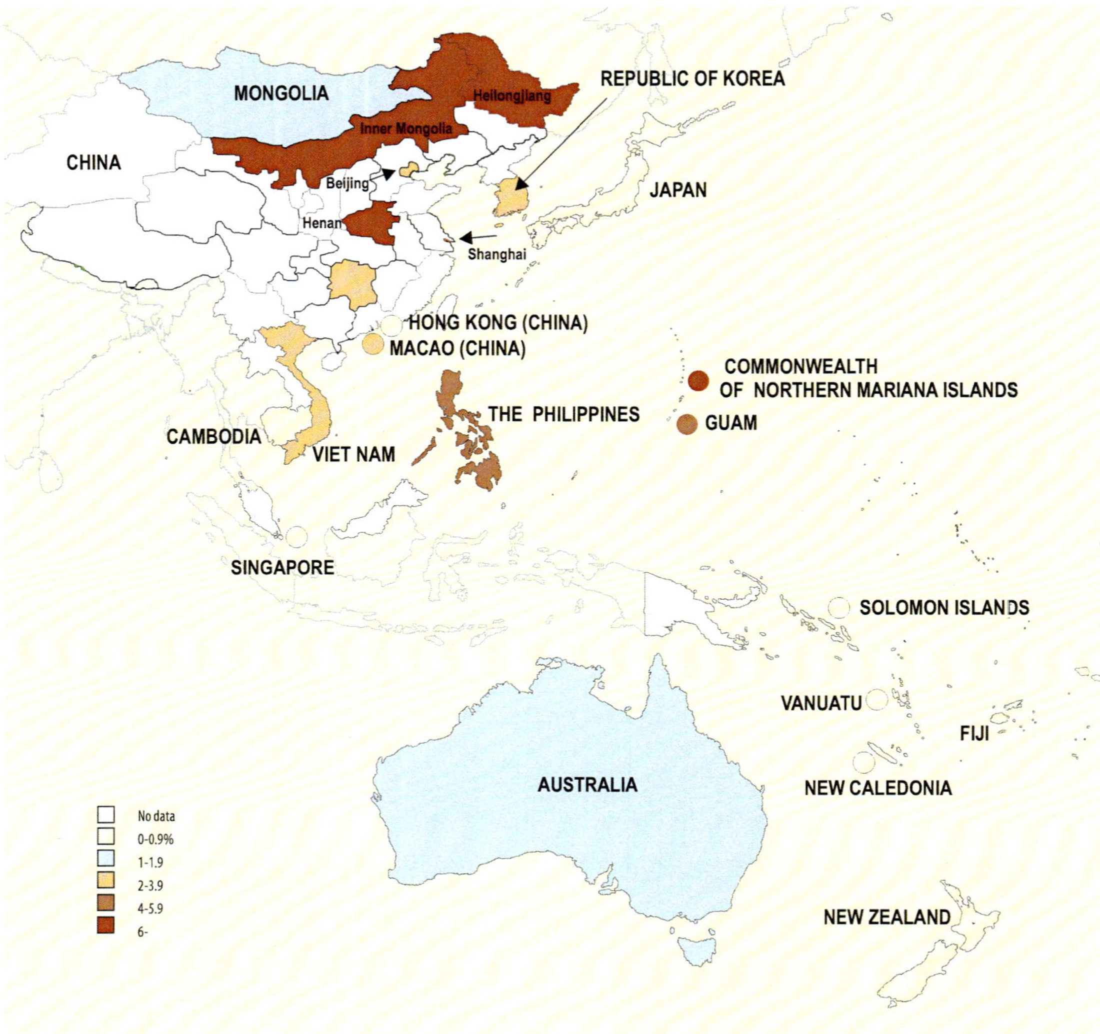


* In the map, the data from Australia, Fiji, Guam, New Caledonia and Solomon Islands indicate new and retreatment cases combined. Only data on new cases are available for the Commonwealth of the Northern Mariana Islands and Vanuatu.

The boundaries shown and the designations used on this map do not imply the expression of any opinion whatsoever on the part of the World Health Organization concerning the legal status of any country, territory, city or area or of its authorities, or concerning the delimitation of its frontiers or boundaries. White lines on maps represent approximate border lines for which there may not yet be full agreement. 

**Figure 10.** Geographic distribution of MDR-TB among retreatment cases by country and area in the Region and by province in China, 2000–2008

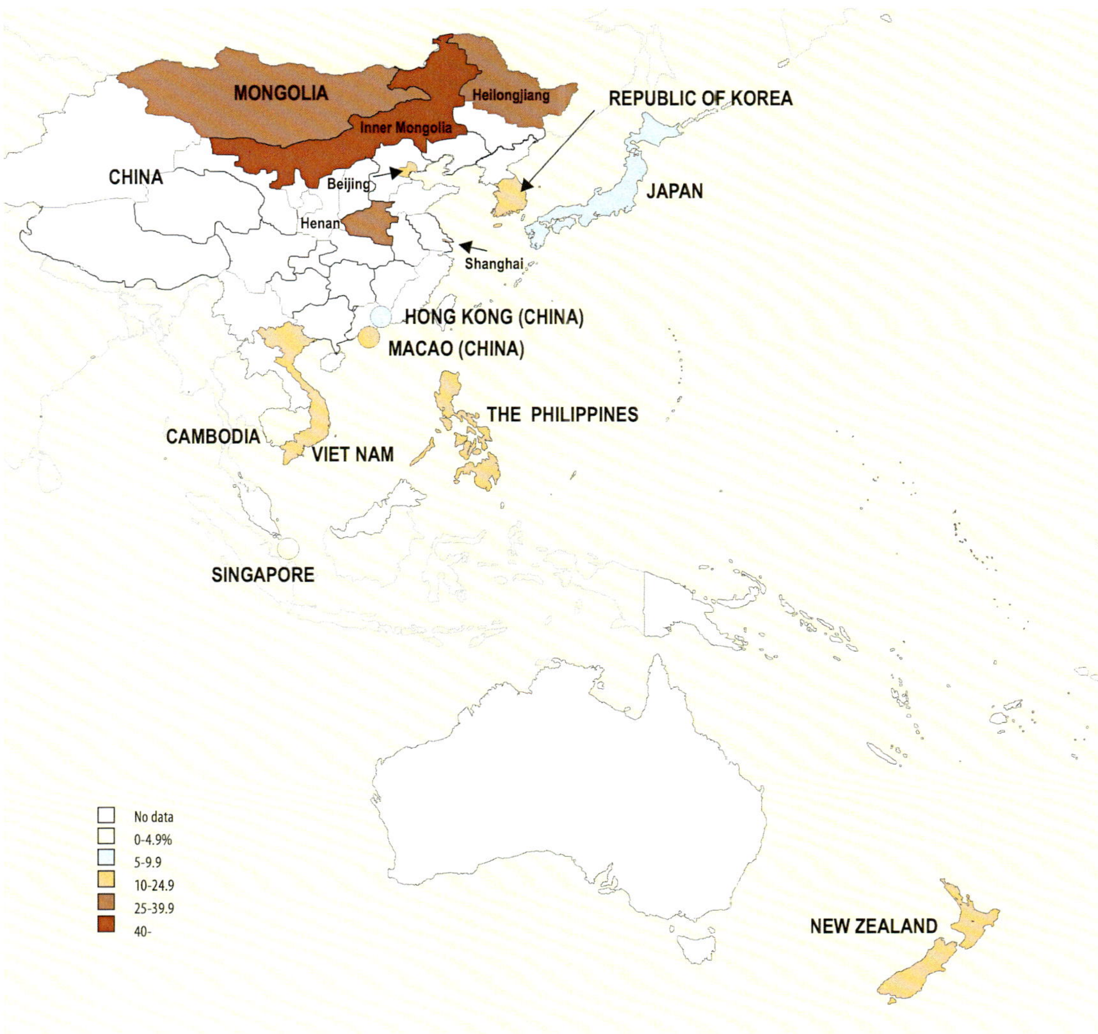


As of 2008, all countries with an intermediate burden of TB except for Brunei Darussalam have conducted DRS. The prevalence of resistance to first line anti-TB drugs is low, except for Macao (China) and Republic of Korea (Table 6).

There are several countries and areas that have reported more than three data points between 1994 and 2008. Figure 11 shows the trend of the proportion of MDR-TB among combined or new cases and the trend of the notification rate of all forms of TB in selected countries in the Region during that period. Hong Kong (China) and Japan reported statistically significant decreasing trends in MDR-TB among new (Hong Kong [China]) or combined (Japan) cases at faster rates than the decline in TB notifications. The trends in MDR-TB declined at 13% and 16% per year while that of all forms of TB declined by 3% and 5% per year in Hong Kong (China) and Japan, respectively. Singapore showed a slight decrease in the prevalence of MDR-TB among new TB cases; however, the numbers were small.

Australia and New Zealand with a low TB prevalence show a fluctuating proportion of MDR-TB over time, possibly because their overall burden of TB is low and the absolute numbers of MDR-TB cases reported in the countries are small. The Republic of Korea has shown a gradual but steadily increasing statistically significant trend in MDR-TB among new cases in five periodic surveys while it showed a relatively stable trend in the TB notification rate, partly because of an expansion of the national surveillance system into the private sector.

**Figure 11.** Trends of proportion of MDR-TB and notification rates of all forms of TB in selected countries and areas in the Region, 1994–2008

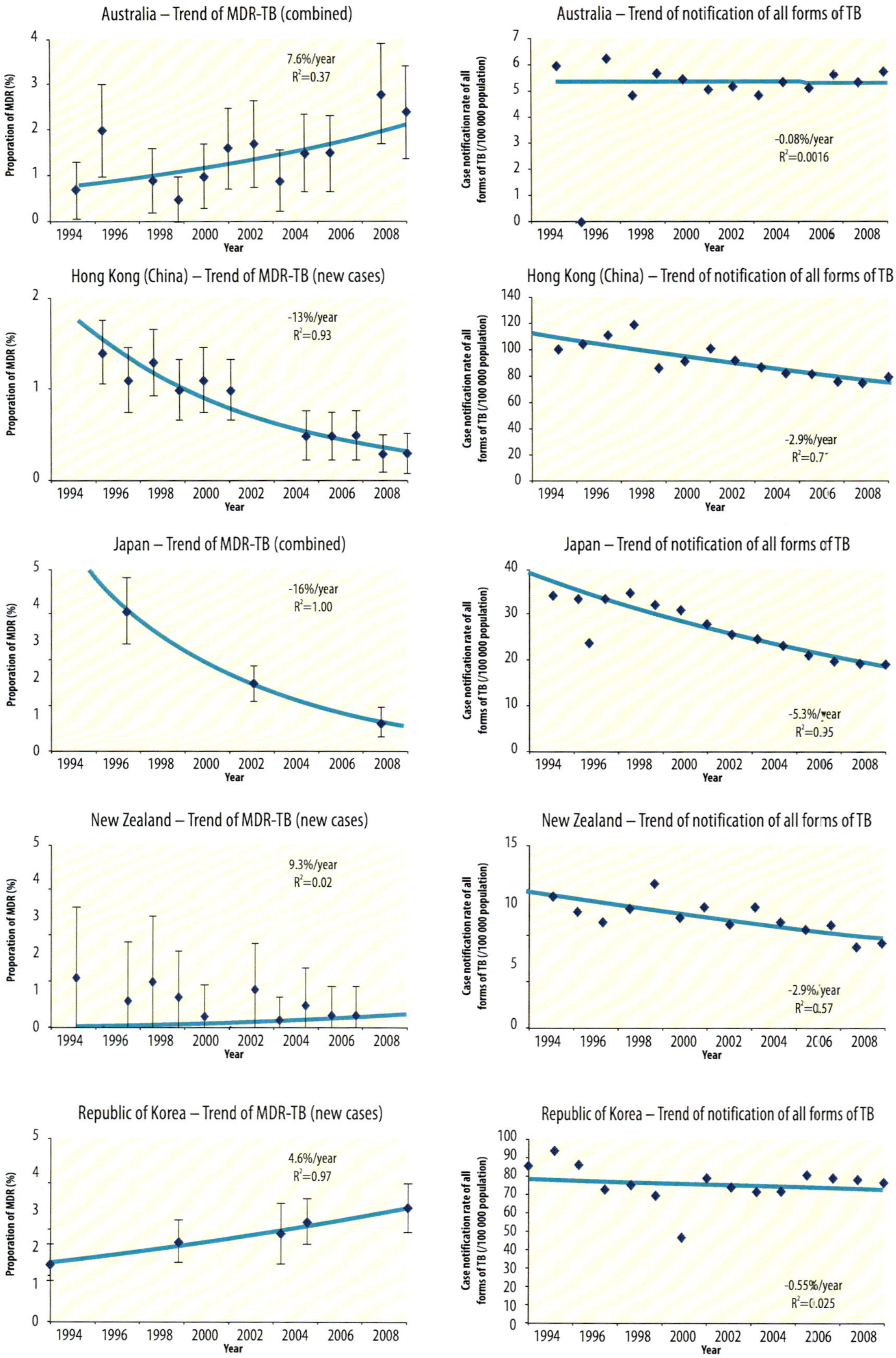

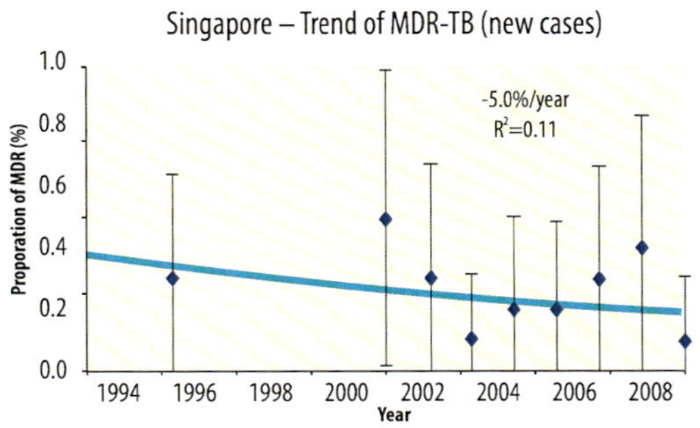


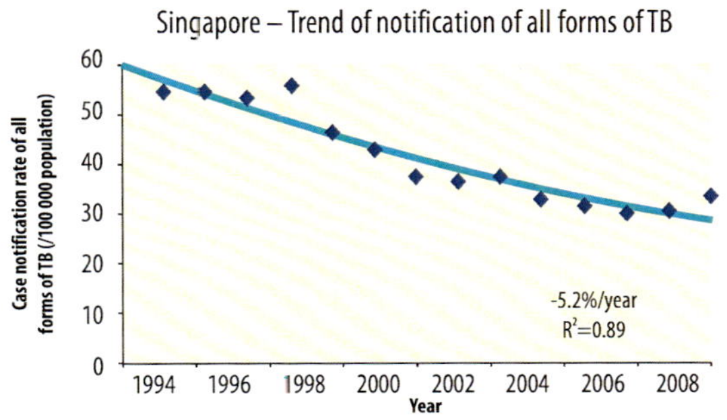


Based on the overall case management data in 2008, however, 1198 new patients and 5734 retreatment patients were reported with available drug susceptibility testing (DST) results in the Region. Of those, 57 (1.0%) new patients and 2301 (38.9%) retreatment patients had MDR-TB. The capacity to detect and treat drug-resistant TB cases remains to be scaled up rapidly in the entire Region, particularly in countries and areas reported to have a high prevalence of MDR-TB.

Currently, information on resistance to second-line anti-TB drugs in the Region is very limited. Between 2006 and 2008, only five countries and areas in the Region -- Australia, Hong Kong (China), Macao (China), Republic of Korea and Singapore -- were able to report data on strains of TB resistance to second-line drugs (Table 7). Hong Kong (China) and the Republic of Korea showed the prevalence of extensively drug-resistant TB (XDR-TB) among MDR-TB strains tested for second-line drugs as n=1 (6.7%) and n=4 (5.1%), respectively, among new cases and n=1 (6.7%) and n=4 (4.4%), respectively, among retreatment cases.

Because the absolute numbers of MDR-TB are low, XDR-TB may not pose a major obstacle for TB control. However, in countries with a high burden of TB where second-line drugs are widely available, such as China and the Philippines, a further assessment of resistance to second-line drugs will be a critical component of designing the appropriate strategy for the management of MDR-TB.

**Table 7.** Extensively drug resistance surveillance, by country and area, 2006–2008

| | | New cases | | | | Retreatment cases | |
|---|---|---|---|---|---|---|---|
| Country and area | Surveillance year | No. of MDR-TB strains tested for second-line anti TB drugs | Resistant to any quino-lones (%) | Resistant to second line injectable agents (%) | XDR-TB (%) | No. of MDR-TB strains tested for second-line anti TB drugs | XDR-TB (%) |
| Australia* | 2007 | 24 | 4.2 | 4.2 | 0 | - | - |
| Hong Kong (China) | 2007–2008 | 15 | 20.0 | 13.3 | 6.7 | 15 | 6.7 |
| Macao (China) | 2008 | 5 | 0 | 0 | 0 | 2 | 0 |
| Republic of Korea | 2008 | 79 | 16.5 | 10.1 | 5.1 | 90 | 4.4 |
| Singapore | 2006–2008 | 7 | 0 | 0 | 0 | 7 | 0 |

No. = number; XDR-TB = extensively drug resistant TB
*Combined new and retreatment cases

**Figure 12.** Estimated percentage of MDR-TB among new (left) and previously treated (right) cases in countries with a high burden of TB, 2008

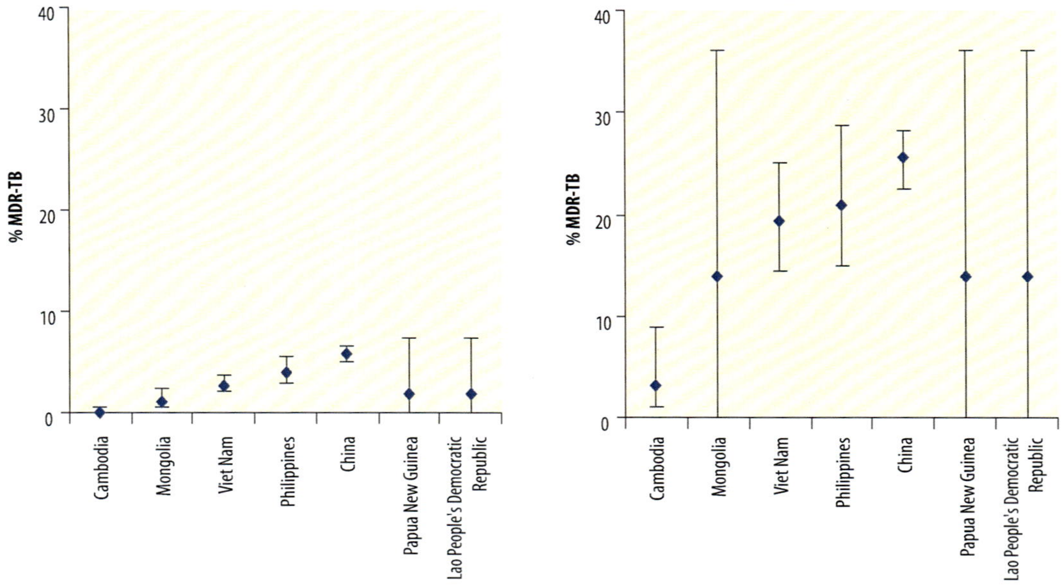


MDR-TB = multidrug-resistant TB
Vertical lines represent 95% confidence intervals of the estimates.
Estimates derived from DRS (Cambodia, China, Mongolia, the Philippines and Viet Nam) and modelling (Lao People's Democratic Republic and Papua New Guinea ).

Overall, there were about 120 000 estimated cases of MDR-TB (primary and acquired[5]) arising in 2008 in the Region, which accounted for about 27% of the estimated global number of MDR-TB. Methods to derive estimates of the MDR-TB burden were explained in Annex 3. The distribution of the estimated proportion of TB cases with MDR-TB in seven countries with a high burden of TB in the Region is shown in Figure 12. Cambodia, China, the Philippines and Viet Nam are estimated to be accounting for 97% of MDR-TB in the Region. The more detailed distribution of the estimated proportions of TB cases with MDR-TB and the absolute number of MDR-TB by country is given in Annex 9.

## 2.6 TB-HIV

### 2.6.1 Surveillance data on HIV in TB cases

HIV infection fuels the TB epidemic, particularly in countries and areas with a high burden of TB, because it reduces cell-mediated immunity and is an important risk factor for the onset of TB. The annual risk of developing active TB in a coinfected person ranges from 5%–15%, depending on the degree of immuno-suppression. In the past 10–15 years, TB case numbers have increased by 300%–400% in high HIV-prevalence countries. To a lesser extent, TB-HIV coinfection also affects some countries and areas in the Region.

The overall percentage of TB patients tested for HIV in the Region remained low with 11% of all notified cases. However, the figure substantially increased in 2008 from 3% and 9% in 2006 and 2007, respectively. Across the 23 reporting countries and areas, HIV testing of 152 468 TB patients led to the identification of 10 551 HIV-positive cases, representing 6.9% of all tested TB cases (Table 8) and 22% of the estimated burden of incident HIV-TB.

---

5 Previously treated cases may have acquired MDR-TB during the course of treatment (numbers estimated under the term acquired MDR-TB) or may have been infected with an MDR-TB strain in the first place. Primary MDR-TB among retreatment cases are counted among MDR-TB among new and relapse cases but are not counted again among retreatment cases.

**Table 8.** Surveillance data on HIV in TB cases in selected countries and areas in the Region, 2008

| Country and area | TB cases notified (new and relapse) | Tested for HIV | | Positive for HIV | |
|---|---|---|---|---|---|
| | | No. | (%) | No. | (%) |
| Brunei Darussalam | 223 | 223 | 100 | - | |
| Cambodia | 38 927 | 21 523 | 55 | 3309 | 15 |
| China | 975 821 | 81 682 | 8 | 2848 | 3 |
| Hong Kong (China) | 5544 | 4121 | 74 | 48 | 1 |
| Japan | 24 181 | 13 777 | 57 | 67 | 0.5 |
| Lao People's Democratic Republic | 4048 | 557 | 14 | 221 | 40 |
| Macao (China) | 359 | 376* | 105 | 1 | 0.3 |
| Malaysia | 17 144 | 14 726 | 86 | 1819 | 12 |
| Mongolia | 4490 | 1296 | 29 | 1 | 0.1 |
| Papua New Guinea | 13 984 | 582 | 4 | - | |
| Philippines | 139 603 | 1069 | 1 | - | |
| Viet Nam | 97 772 | 11 332 | 12 | 2210 | 20 |
| **Western Pacific Region** | **1 363 480** | **152 468** | **11** | **10 551** | **7** |

* The definition of TB cases tested for HIV may differ in each country from that of notified TB cases (new and relapse) because the numbers may include other retreatment cases than relapse

- = data unavailable, No. = number, % = percentage

**Figure 13.** National prevalence surveys on TB-HIV coinfection, Cambodia, 2003–2009

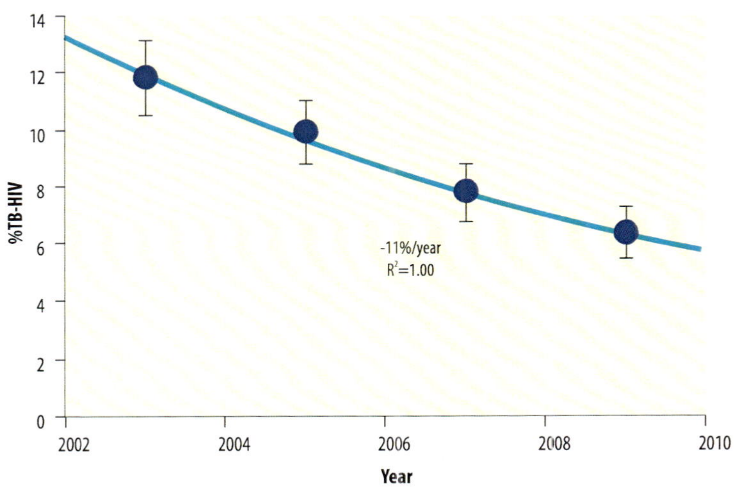


In Cambodia, four national surveys of HIV prevalence in TB patients showed a statistically significant decline from 11.8% in 2003 to 6.3% in 2009 (Figure 13), which is much lower than the routine surveillance data shown in Table 8 above. The reason may well be explained by the health staff's biased tendency to test TB cases with a severe general condition suggestive of AIDS or from risk groups. In Malaysia, HIV and TB cases share important risk factors and the two epidemics are highly concentrated in similar populations (i.e. injecting drug users [IDUs]).

In some areas in Papua New Guinea, the prevalence of HIV among TB patients was considerably higher than previously estimated. Data from sentinel surveillance centres in three major health facilities in Port Moresby, Goroka and Lae showed that 12% to 19% of TB cases were HIV coinfected in 2003.[6] Another report on the routine surveillance data showed 117 and 1134 TB cases were tested for HIV in 2007 and 2008,

6 National Department of Health, Papua New Guinea, 2006.

respectively, of which 17 (15%) and 116 (10%), respectively, were HIV-positive.[7] Sentinel surveillance in 2008 also showed a 19% TB-HIV coinfection rate.[8] In Ho Chi Minh City, Viet Nam, the prevalence had significantly increased from 1.5% between 1997 and 1998 to 9.0% between 2001 and 2002.[9] The prevalence remains high at 7.7% in selected districts of Ho Chi Minh City between 2006 and 2007.[10]

### 2.6.2 Estimated prevalence of HIV among the general population and new TB cases

Papua New Guinea has a generalized HIV epidemic (HIV prevalence >1% of the national population) with an estimated 1.5% (low–high estimate: 1.4–1.6) of the adult population (15–49 years old) infected with HIV in 2007.[11] Cambodia used to have a generalized HIV epidemic. However, the prevalence is estimated to have decreased from a peak of 2.0% in 1998 down to below 0.8% (low–high estimate: 0.7–0.9) in adults (15–49 years old) in 2007. In other countries and areas in the Western Pacific Region, the prevalence of HIV in adults has remained stable or slightly has increased between 2001 and 2007.

The prevalence of HIV in incident TB cases was estimated to be highest in Cambodia (15%) followed by Malaysia (12%) and Papua New Guinea (3.8%) and Viet Nam (3.8%). The prevalence was estimated to be low in Mongolia (0.15%) and in the Philippines (0.26%) (Figure 14). In terms of absolute numbers of HIV coinfection in incident TB cases, however, China was most affected (22 000) because of its huge population, followed by Cambodia (11 000) and Viet Nam (6 000).

**Figure 14.** Estimated HIV prevalence in new TB cases in selected countries and areas in the Region, 2008

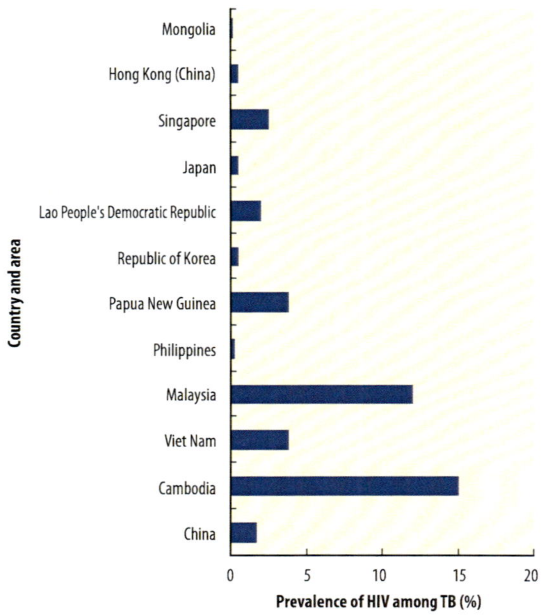


**(a) Prevalence of HIV among TB (%)**

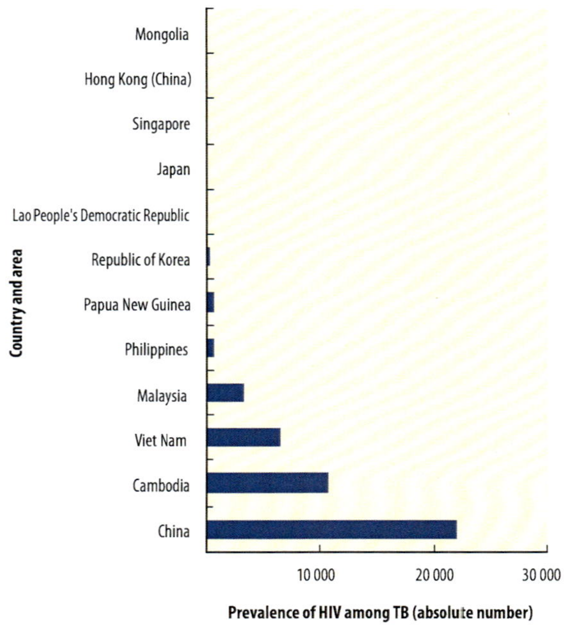


**(b) Prevalence of HIV among TB (absolute number)**

In all countries and areas in the Region, HIV prevalence in new TB cases is consistently higher than the prevalence of HIV in the general adult population (Figure 15).

---

7 National TB Programme case notification report, 2009, Papua New Guinea.

8 Unpublished data, Sentinel survey 2008, National TB Programme, National Department of Health, Papua New Guinea

9 Tran NB *et al.* HIV and tuberculosis in Ho Chi Minh City, Viet Nam, 1997–2002. *Emerging Infectious Diseases*, 2007:13:1463–1469.

10 Data presented at the Meeting on the Revised TB-HIV Co-Infection Framework for the Western Pacific Region held in February 2008.

11 2008 Report on the global AIDS epidemic, UNAIDS/WHO, 2008. (http://www.unaids.org/en/KnowledgeCentre/HIVData/GlobalReport/2008/2008_Global_report.asp)

**Figure 15.** Estimated prevalence of HIV in new TB cases against prevalence of HIV in adults in selected countries and areas in the Region, 2008

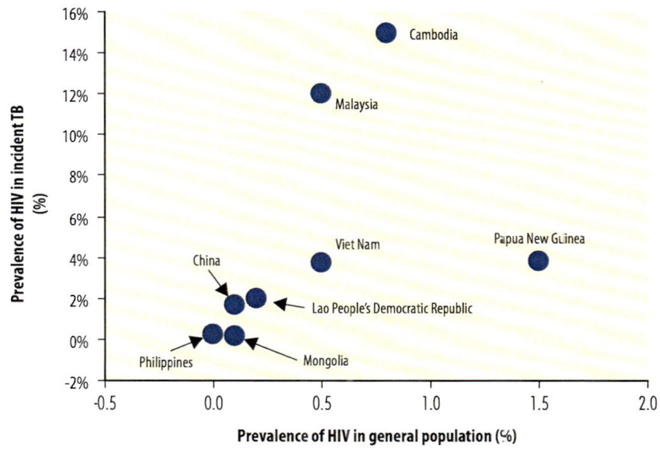

# 3 TB Control

## 3.1 Case detection and trend

By the end of 2007, directly observed treatment, short-course (DOTS) coverage had reached 100% coverage in the Region. Since 2008 WHO no longer collected information about DOTS coverage.

In 2005, the Region reached the global and regional target of detecting 70% of the estimated new sputum-positive TB cases and has sustained high case detection rates since then (Figure 16).

**Figure 16.** Trends in DOTS coverage and case detection in smear-positive cases in the Region, 1995–2008

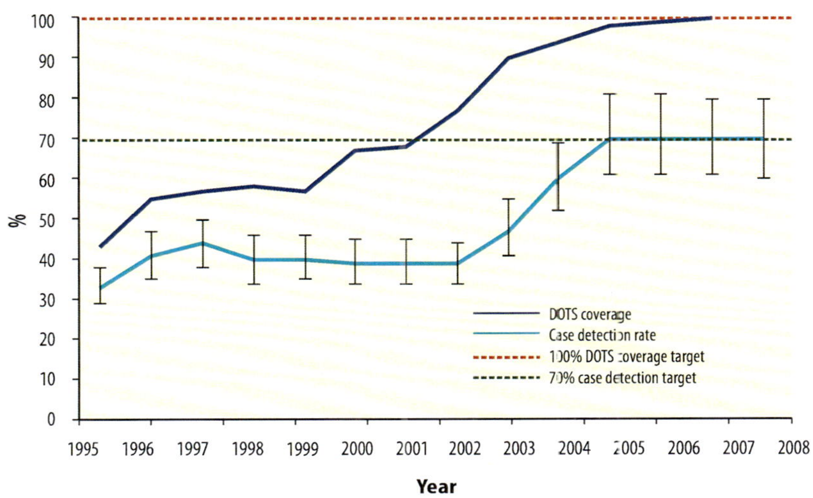


Data on DOTS coverage is only available until 2007.
DOTS = directly observed treatment, short-course
Case detection rate was calculated by dividing annual new smear-positive notifications under DOTS with estimated annual new smear-positive incidence.
The error bar shows the low and high estimates for each year.

## 3.2 Treatment outcomes

The Region continued to observe treatment success rates beyond the target of 85%. Of 0.7 million new pulmonary smear-positive cases registered for treatment in 2007, treatment success has been remarkably high, with 92% overall. Across the Region, 20 countries and areas reached the 85% treatment success target. Among the countries with a high burden of TB, the treatment success rates was highest in China and Cambodia (94%) followed by Viet Nam and Lao People's Democratic Republic (92%) and Mongolia (89%) and the Philippines (89%). The treatment success rate of Papua New Guinea was lowest with 39%, with almost half of the 2007 cohort unevaluated (Figure 17).

**Figure 17.** Treatment outcomes for new smear-positive cases registered in 2007 in countries with a high burden of TB in the Region
DOTS: directly observed treatment, short-course. Numbers in bars are treatment success rates.

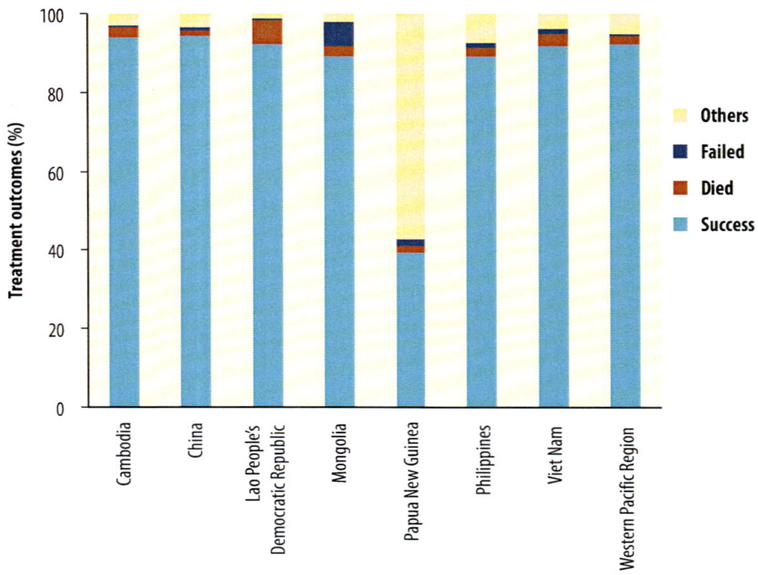


Overall, unfavourable treatment outcomes were reported for 8% of new smear-positive cases and 14% of retreatment smear-positive cases of the 2007 cohort. About one quarter of those with unfavourable outcomes died. Failures and defaulters accounted for 28% of unfavourable outcomes among new smear-positive cases and 35% among retreatment smear-positive cases (Figure 18). Transfer-out accounted for 36% of unfavourable treatment outcomes. About 10% of cases could not be evaluated in both cohorts. The cases reported under transfer-out can have any of the other treatment outcomes, but detailed information is not available because follow-up outcomes are not recorded in the TB registers.

**Figure 18.** Unfavourable outcomes among new smear-positive cases and retreatment smear-positive cases registered in 2007 in the Region

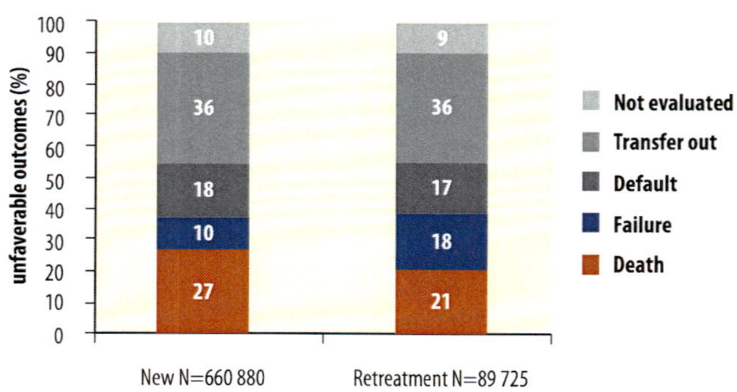


Number in each segment indicates the respective proportion of treatment outcome .

## 3.3 Laboratory capacity

In the seven countries with a high burden of TB in the Region, there were 6981 TB laboratories performing acid-fast bacilli (AFB) smear microscopy in 2008, 6460 (93%) of which participated in external quality assessment (EQA) programmes. In five of these countries—Cambodia, China, the Lao People's Democratic Republic, Mongolia and Viet Nam—almost all sputum smear microscopy centres participated in EQA activities and over 80% of these laboratories showed satisfactory results in EQA (Table 9). Between 2007 and 2008, the proportion of laboratories participating in EQA programmes decreased significantly from 100% to 81% in the Philippines. But in Papua New Guinea, the number of sputum smear microscopy laboratories increased from 70 to 111, whereas the proportion of those participating in EQA decreased from 49% to 36%.

**Table 9.** External quality assessment of sputum smear microscopy in countries with a high burden of TB in the Region, 2008

| Country | No. of smear microscopy laboratories | Laboratories included in EQA (%) | Laboratories included in EQA | | | Laboratories showed satisfactory** result in EQA | |
|---|---|---|---|---|---|---|---|
| | | | No. | % | % Change from 2007* | No. | % |
| Cambodia | 202 | 1.4 | 202 | 100 | 8 | 166 | 82 |
| China | 3294 | 0.2 | 3294 | 100 | 0 | 3280 | 100 |
| Lao People's Democratic Republic | 155 | 2.6 | 154 | 99 | 0 | 145 | 94 |
| Mongolia | 36 | 1.4 | 36 | 100 | 0 | 31 | 86 |
| Papua New Guinea | 111 | 1.7 | 40 | 36 | -26 | 23 | 58 |
| Philippines | 2374 | 2.6 | 1925 | 81 | -19 | 1791 | 93 |
| Viet Nam | 809 | 0.9 | 809 | 100 | - | 769 | 95 |

EQA = external quality assessment; No. = number; labs = laboratories; pop. = population;
- = no data in 2007 report and thus unable to compare
* Defined as the proportion of laboratories included in EQA in 2008 divided by that in 2007 expressed in percentage.
** Defined as showing either high false-positive (HFP) or high false-negative (HFN) in a round of EQA (i.e. normally a year of four quarters)

In seven countries with a high burden of TB in the Region, there were 666 laboratories capable of performing AFB culture and 117 capable of performing DST for first-line anti-TB drugs in 2008. Of these, 628 and 109, respectively, were located in China. All seven countries with a high burden of TB, except for the Lao People's Democratic Republic, have at least one laboratory performing culture and DST. Overall, the number of laboratories capable of performing culture and DST is insufficient in the Region, particularly in the Lao People's Democratic Republic, the Philippines and Viet Nam (DST facility only), given the occurrence of MDR-TB and TB-HIV coinfection and given the need to detect and treat cases under such conditions.

**Table 10.** Laboratory services in countries with a high burden of TB in the Region, 2008

| Country | Population (thousand) | Culture | | DST | |
|---|---|---|---|---|---|
| | | No. of labs | /5 mil. pop | No. of labs | /10 mil. pop |
| Cambodia | 14 562 | 3 | 1.0 | 1 | 0.7 |
| China | 1 337 411 | 628 | 2.4 | 109 | 0.8 |
| Lao People's Democratic Republic | 5859 | 0 | 0.0 | 0 | 0.0 |
| Mongolia | 2641 | 1 | 1.9 | 1 | 3.8 |
| Papua New Guinea | 6577 | 1 | 0.8 | 1 | 1.5 |
| Philippines | 90 348 | 3 | 0.2 | 3 | 0.3 |
| Viet Nam | 87 096 | 30 | 1.7 | 2 | 0.2 |

No. = number; pop. = population; DST = drug susceptibility testing; mil = million
To provide cultures for diagnosis of paediatric, extrapulmonary and smear-negative HIV-infected TB cases, as well as DST for retreatment and failure cases, most countries and areas will need one culture facility per 5 million population and one DST facility per 10 million population. However, for countries and areas with large populations, one laboratory for culture and DST in each major administrative area (e.g. province) may be sufficient.

A network of laboratories was established in conjunction with the Global Project on Antituberculosis Drug Resistance Surveillance (see section 2.5 Drug resistance) and named the supranational laboratory network (SRLN). The SRLN participates in annual proficiency testing and has a mandate to assist national reference laboratories in laboratory assessments: in proficiency testing, quality assurance of results from drug resistance surveys and other technical guidance as necessary. There are six supranational reference laboratories in the Region (Table 11).

**Table 11.** Supranational reference laboratories (SRLs) in the Region and countries and areas to which an SRL provide support

| Supranational reference laboratory | Countries and Areas |
|---|---|
| Institute of Medical and Veterinary Science (IMVS), Adelaide, Australia | Viet Nam, Pacific island countries and areas |
| Korean Institute of Tuberculosis (KIT), Seoul, the Republic of Korea | The Philippines |
| Queensland Mycobacterium Reference Laboratory (QMRL), Brisbane, Australia | Papua New Guinea, Pacific island countries and areas |
| Research Institute of Tuberculosis (RIT), Tokyo, Japan | Cambodia, Mongolia, the Philippines |
| Tuberculosis Reference Laboratory, Department of Health, Hong Kong (China) | China, Lao People's Democratic Republic |
| The Centers for Disease Control and Prevention (CDC), Atlanta, United States of America, through Diagnostic Laboratory Services, Inc.*, Hawaii, United States of America | American Samoa, Guam, the Commonwealth of the Northern Mariana Islands, the Marshall Islands, the Federated States of Micronesia, Palau |

*Not a member of the supranational laboratory network

In the Pacific island countries and areas, a TB laboratory network was established in 2004 in collaboration with the Institute of Medical and Veterinary Science, Adelaide, Australia; the Queensland Mycobacterium Reference Laboratory, Brisbane, Australia; the Pacific Paramedical Training Centre (PPTC), Wellington, New Zealand; the Secretariat of the Pacific Community (SPC); the Centers for Disease Control and Prevention in the United States of America; and WHO.

The network is called the Pacific TB Laboratory (PaTLab) Initiative. The primary objective of the PaTLab is to improve the quality of sputum smear-microscopy by application of EQA and to expand surveillance for drug-resistant TB. The PaTLab coordinates EQA of sputum smear-microscopy, including panel testing, blind rechecking and onsite visits. The PaTLab has initiated DRS in some Pacific island countries, as described in Section 2.5. The PaTLab has contributed significantly to the quality improvement of TB laboratory services in the Pacific island countries.

# 4 Profiles of countries with a high burden of TB in the Region

This section highlights epidemiologic indicators for seven countries with a high burden of TB in the Region. Overall, these countries accounted for 94% of the regional estimated incident cases. The plans of activities for MDR-TB control of each country are also included.

## 4.1 Cambodia

The final results of the 2008 population census show that the Cambodian population has increased by 1.96 million over the last 10 years from 11.4 million in 1998 to 13.4 million in 2008. However, data for this report are still based on the United Nations Population Division's estimate of 14.562 million for 2008. This estimate is expected to be revised according to the census conducted in 2008. The population density of the country increased from 64 to 75 people per square kilometre and the annual growth rate declined from 2.5% in 1998 to 1.5% in 2008. The median age is 20, with the proportion of those under 15 years old at 37%. The population sex ratio (males per 100 females) was 95 in 2005. About 20% of the population lived in urban areas in 2006.

Cambodia is one of 22 countries worldwide with a high burden of TB. It has the highest estimated incidence, prevalence and mortality rates in the Region. Although the national HIV prevalence in adults and HIV prevalence among incident TB cases has declined substantially in recent years,[12] Cambodia remains affected by a significant TB-HIV epidemic. Drug-resistant TB is starting to emerge among retreatment cases.

The main achievements of the NTP include sustaining treatment success above 85% for over a decade, improving access to TB services through community-based DOTS and expanding TB-HIV collaborative activities to an increasing number of provinces. Major challenges include strengthening the quality-assured laboratory network and increasing laboratory capacity, addressing infection control issues, increasing case detection and improving the motivation of staff.

The NTP planned to conduct a second nationwide prevalence survey in 2010, with financial support from the Japan International Cooperation Agency (JICA), the Global Fund to Fight AIDS, Tuberculosis and Malaria and the United States of America Agency for International Development (USAID) through the Tuberculosis Control Assistance Program (TBCAP) and technical support from WHO and the Research Institute of Tuberculosis (RIT).

12 See section 2.6 on TB-HIV.

**Figure 19.** Cambodia

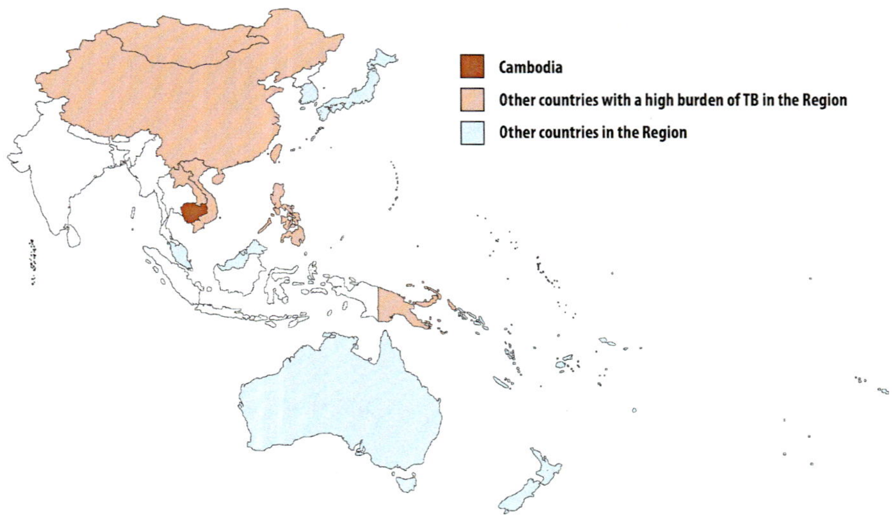


**Table 12.** Key indicators of TB control, Cambodia, 2008

| | |
|---|---|
| Population (thousands) | 14 562 |
| TB burden (2008 estimate) | |
| Incidence (all forms/100 000 population) | 490 [390–590] |
| Incidence (ss+/100 000 population) | 240 [190–290] |
| Prevalence (all forms/100 000 population) | 680 [400–1100] |
| Mortality (deaths/100 000 population) | 79 [33–150] |
| Prevalence of HIV in adult incident TB cases (%) | 15 [12–18] |
| New multidrug-resistant TB cases (%)* | 0.0 |
| Previously treated multidrug-resistant TB cases (%)* | 3.1 |

*Data from the DRS conducted in 2001

**Table 13.** DOTS implementation, Cambodia, 2008

| | |
|---|---|
| Number of notified cases (new and relapse) | 38 927 |
| Notification rate (new and relapse/100 000 population) | 267 |
| Notification rate (new ss+/100 000 population) | 136 |
| Case detection (new and relapse, %) Best [Low-High estimates] | 55 [45–68] |
| Treatment success (2007 cohort new ss+, %) | 94 |

## Surveillance and epidemiology

Since 2000, the case notification rate for all forms of TB has increased significantly from 148 to 267 per 100 000 population (Figure 20, trend +5.4% per year). However, the case notification rate of new smear-positive cases has remained almost stable since 2002, ranging from 130 to 149 per 100 000 population (trend +0.2% per year).

**Figure 20.** Trend of case notification rates (all forms of TB and smear-positive), Cambodia, 2000–2008

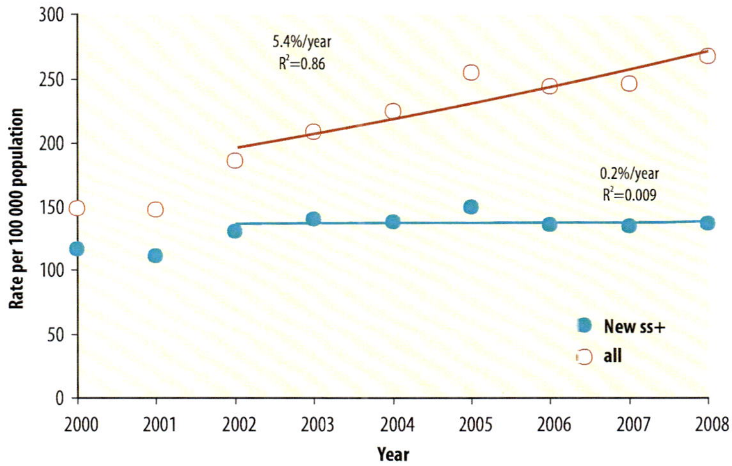


**Figure 21.** Geographical distribution of notification rates of all forms of TB, Cambodia, 2008

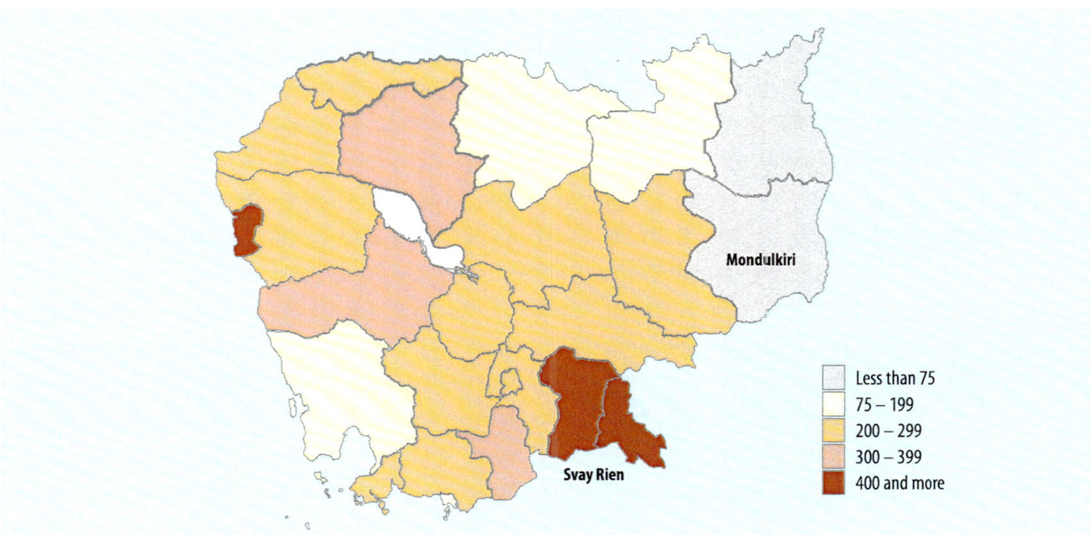


The notification rate of all forms of TB varies among provinces and remains highest in Svay Rieng at 460/100 000 population, while it is lowest in Mondulkiri (56/100 000 population) (Figure 21). Provincial figures are available in Annex 8.

**Figure 22.** Distribution of forms of TB among new cases, Cambodia, 2003–2008

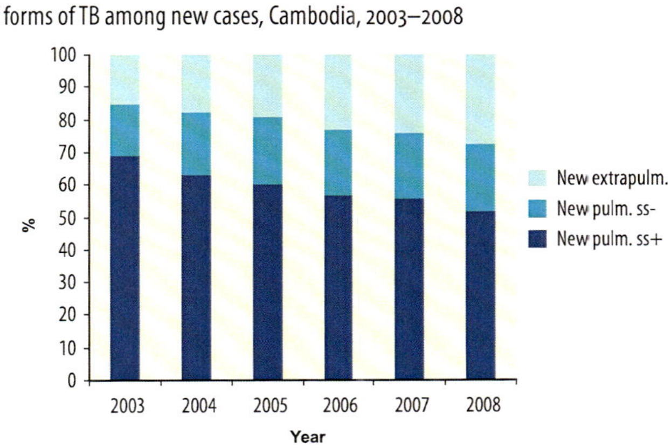


extrapulm. = extrapulmonary; pulm. = pulmonary; ss- or ss+ = sputum smear negative or positive

The distribution of forms of TB among new cases notified between 2003 and 2008 is shown in Figure 22. The proportion of smear-positive cases gradually has decreased from 69% to 52%, while that of extrapulmonary TB cases has increased from 15% to 28%. The proportion of smear-negative cases remained stable with a range of 16%-20%.

**Table 14.** Trend of DOTS performance indicators, Cambodia, 2000–2008

| | 2000 | 2001 | 2002 | 2003 | 2004 | 2005 | 2006 | 2007 | 2008 |
|---|---|---|---|---|---|---|---|---|---|
| DOTS coverage (%) | 99 | 100 | 100 | 100 | 100 | 100 | 100 | 100 | - |
| Notification rate (new and relapse/100 000 population) | 148 | 147 | 186 | 209 | 225 | 255 | 244 | 246 | 267 |
| Notification rate (new ss+/100 000 population) | 116 | 110 | 130 | 140 | 138 | 150 | 136 | 134 | 136 |
| Case detection rate (new and relapse, %) | 28 | 28 | 36 | 41 | 44 | 51 | 49 | 50 | 55 |
| Treatment success (new ss+, %) | 91 | 92 | 92 | 93 | 91 | 93 | 93 | 94 | - |
| Retreatment success (ss+, %) | 90 | 92 | 89 | 87 | 86 | 76 | 83 | 83 | - |

Cambodia has sustained high treatment success rates in new and retreatment smear-positive cases between 2000 and 2007 (Table 14).

### MDR-TB activities

Cambodia received approval for the enrolment of 130 MDR-TB cases after submitting a Green Light Committee (GLC) application in 2006, through a joint nongovernmental organization (NGO) and the NTP project. In late 2009, 110 patients were treated through these NGO-initiated projects, which are closely implemented with the NTP in existing public health facilities. The NTP and partners plan to further scale up these initiatives and the NTP has submitted a GLC application for 280 patients. The NGO has requested expansion of its cohort for an additional 150 patients.

A technical working group for MDR-TB has been established under the stewardship of the National Center for Tuberculosis and Leprosy Control (CENAT), and with representations from all key partners.

The main challenge relates to strengthening the national and two regional laboratories to perform reliable quality-assured culture and DST services for MDR-TB and necessary funding to scale up the MDR-TB programme for nationwide coverage. The NTP is planning to apply for Global Fund Round 10 in 2010.

The policy on MDR-TB control has been established within the NTP. The summary is shown in Table 15. Table 16 summarizes the country's future plans related to MDR-TB treatment during the period 2009–2014.

**Table 15.** Summary of NTP policy on MDR-TB treatment, Cambodia

| Items | Policy |
|---|---|
| Case finding strategy | Failure to CAT I and II, RAD, relapse, contact with a known MDR-TB case, and nonconverter at month three |
| Source of referral | Public facilities (incl. DOTS clinics, HCs, and national, provincial and district hospitals) |
| Treatment strategy | Standardized (6 Km[Cm]LfxEtoCs[Pas]EZ 18 LfxEtoCs[Pas]EZ) |
| Method of provision of treatment | Partially hospitalized until culture becomes negative and ambulatory for rest of the period |
| Type of treatment supervisor | Home care DOTS by either HCWs or DOT watchers |

CAT = category; RAD = return after default; HCs = health centres; DOT = direct observed treatment; HCWs = health care workers

**Table 16.** Future projections regarding MDR-TB treatment, Cambodia, 2009–2014

| End of | 2009 | 2010 | 2011 | 2012 | 2013 | 2014 |
|---|---|---|---|---|---|---|
| Number of culture facilities to be functional | 3 | 3 | 3 | 5 | 5 | 5 |
| Number of DST facilities to be functional | 1 | 1 | 1 | 1 | 1 | 1 |
| Number of MDR-TB treatment sites to be functional (including hospital- and health centre-based) | 8 | 9 | 12 | 16 | 20 | 24 |
| Number of cases to get DST for diagnosis for MDR-TB | | 200 | 220 | 240 | 400 | 600 |
| Percentage of patients getting DST of total estimated number of smear positive cases | | n/a | n/a | n/a | n/a | n/a |
| Number of MDR-TB cases newly enrolled on treatment | | 100 | 110 | 120 | 200 | 300 |
| Percentage of newly enrolled patients of total estimated number of MDR-TB cases | | 25% | 28% | 30% | 50% | 75% |

n/a = not applicable

## 4.2 China

China is the most populous country in the world with an estimated 1.3 billion citizens. Population growth rates have slowed and life expectancy has risen in recent decades. While life expectancy for children born in China in the 1950s was 46 years, it was over 71 years for those born in 2000. The median age of the population is 31, with the proportion of those under 15 years old at 24%. The population sex ratio (males per 100 females) was 107.7 in 2005. About 88% of the population lived in urban areas in 2006.

China is maintaining an overall high case detection and treatment success rate while accelerating efforts to improve access to health care for all people with TB in order to reduce prevalence and mortality. Capacity-building and activities to improve the quality of data and their analysis (subnational, disaggregated) will contribute to a better understanding and identification of hard-to-reach populations (migrants, ethnic minorities, women, the elderly and populations at risk). China was conducting the third nationwide TB prevalence survey in 2010.

**Figure 23.** China

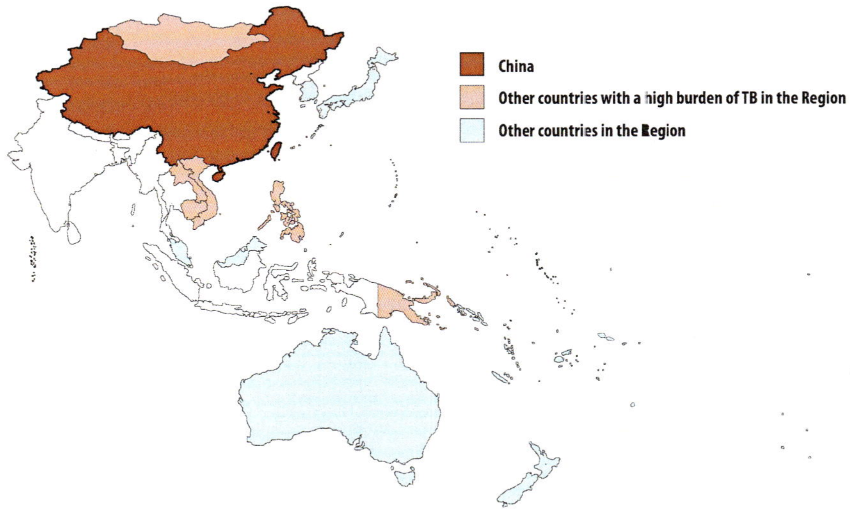


**Table 17.** Key indicators of TB control, China, 2008

| | |
|---|---|
| Population (thousands) | 1 337 411 |
| TB burden (2008 estimate) | |
| Incidence (all forms/100 000 population) | 97 [78–120] |
| Incidence (ss+/100 000 population) | 48 [38–58] |
| Prevalence (all forms/100 000 population) | 88 [31–160] |
| Mortality (deaths/100 000 population) | 12 [4.8–25] |
| Prevalence of HIV in adult incident TB cases (%) | 1.7 [0.23–2.7] |
| New multidrug-resistant TB cases (%)* | 5.7 [4.6–7.1] |
| Previously treated multidrug-resistant TB cases (%)* | 25.6 [21.7–30.0] |

*Data from the DRS conducted in 2007

**Table 18.** DOTS implementation, China, 2008

| | |
|---|---|
| Number of notified cases (new and relapse) | 975 821 |
| Notification rate (new and relapse/100 000 population) | 73 |
| Notification rate (new ss+/100 000 population) | 35 |
| Case detection (new and relapse, %) Best [Low-High estimates] | 75 [62–94] |
| Treatment success (2007 cohort new ss+, %) | 94 |

## Surveillance and epidemiology

Since 2002, case notification rates for all forms of TB and of smear-positive TB have increased significantly from 36 to 73 per 100 000 population and from 15 to 35 per 100 000 population, respectively. However, the notification rate of new smear-positive TB has stabilized at about 35 per 100 000 since 2005 (Figure 24).

**Figure 24.** Trend of case notification rates (all forms of TB and smear-positive), China, 2000–2008

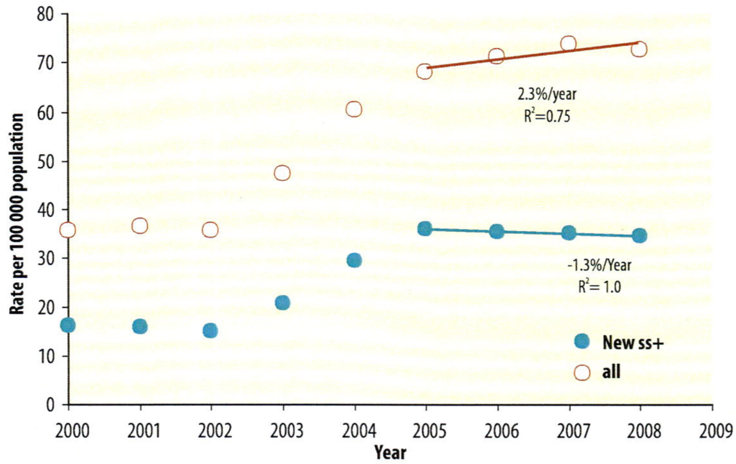


**Figure 25.** Geographical distribution of notification rates of all forms of TB, China, 2008

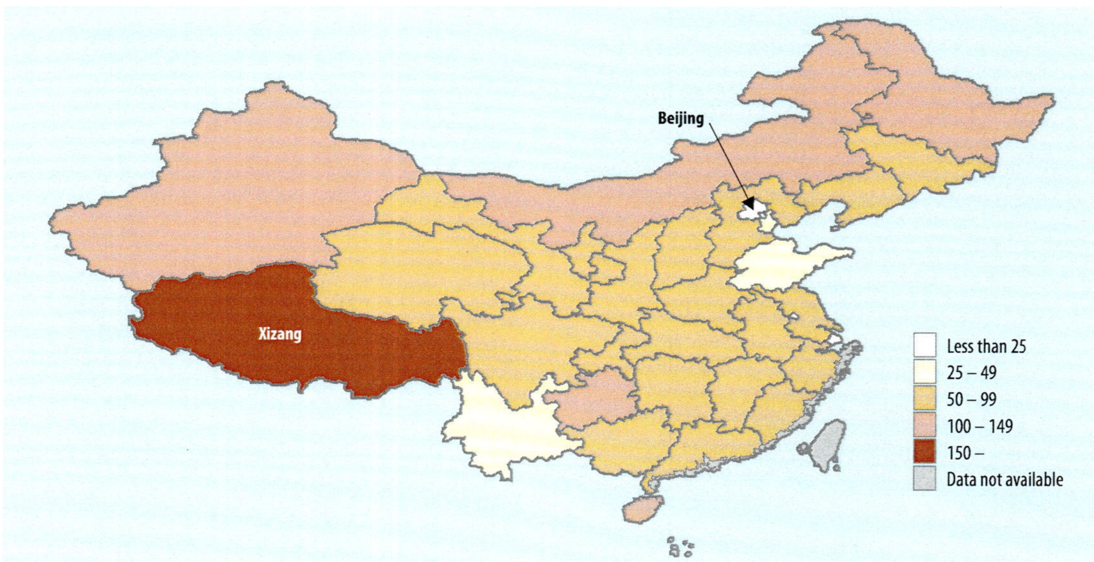


The boundaries shown and the designations used on this map do not imply the expression of any opinion whatsoever on the part of the World Health Organization concerning the legal status of any country, territory, city or area or of its authorities, or concerning the delimitation of its frontiers or boundaries. Black lines on maps represent approximate border lines for which there may not yet be full agreement. 

The notification rates of all forms of TB vary greatly among provinces: it is highest in Xizang (160/100 000 population) and lowest in Beijing (15/100 000 population) (Figure 25). Provincial figures are available in Annex 8.

**Figure 26.** Distribution of forms of TB among new cases, China, 2003–2008

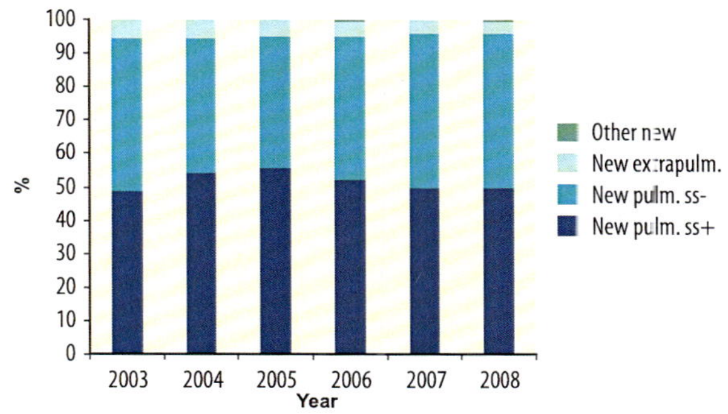


extrapulm. = extrapulmonary; pulm. = pulmonary; ss- or ss+ = sputum smear negative or positive

The distribution of forms of TB among new cases notified between 2003 and 2008 is shown in Figure 26. The proportion of smear-positive cases increased from 49% in 2003 to 56% in 2005 and then declined to 50% in 2008. The proportion of smear-negative cases decreased from 45% in 2003 to 39% in 2005 and then increased again to 46% in 2008. The proportion of extrapulmonary cases gradually decreased from 6% in 2003 to 4% in 2008. The country sustained high treatment success rates between 2000 and 2007 (Table 19).

**Table 19.** Trend of DOTS performance indicators, China, 2000–2008

| | 2000 | 2001 | 2002 | 2003 | 2004 | 2005 | 2006 | 2007 | 2008 |
|---|---|---|---|---|---|---|---|---|---|
| DOTS coverage (%) | 68 | 68 | 78 | 91 | 96 | 100 | 100 | 100 | - |
| Notification rate (new and relapse/100 000 population) | 36 | 37 | 36 | 47 | 61 | 68 | 71 | 74 | 73 |
| Notification rate (new ss+/100 000 population) | 16 | 16 | 15 | 21 | 29 | 36 | 35 | 35 | 35 |
| Case detection rate (new and relapse, %) | 34 | 35 | 35 | 46 | 60 | 68 | 72 | 75 | 75 |
| Treatment success (new ss+, %) | 95 | 96 | 93 | 94 | 94 | 94 | 94 | 94 | - |
| Retreatment success (ss+, %) | 89 | 93 | 88 | 89 | 89 | 90 | 89 | 89 | - |

## MDR-TB activities

Currently, programmatic management of drug-resistant TB (PMDT) is implemented in some provinces in China, funded by Global Fund Round 5 and 7, and other sources, in which about 40 000 MDR-TB cases are expected to be detected and treated by 2015. China has created the national framework for PMDT, the national action plan for PMDT and a series of technical manuals to expedite the scaling-up of PMDT. A stepwise approach will be adopted starting from a central level pilot phase, then to a preliminary scale-up phase, then to a rapid scale-up phase and followed by a full coverage phase. At the current stage, the Global Fund project plays a very important role in piloting PMDT.

By applying the Global Fund Round 9 project and piloting the Bill & Melinda Gates Foundation demonstrative project, China will implement the "enhanced model for PMDT". The target group for MDR-TB screening will be widened from high-risk groups to all sputum smear-positive cases. The laboratory testing method will be shifted from conventional solid-media culture and DST to rapid molecular techniques based on line probe assay (LPA).

From a management aspect, China is practising and will expand two optional patient-centred approaches for MDR-TB management, which are:
Basic model:

- Prefecture: case finding, hospitalization and treatment
- County: suspect screening, referral and outpatient management
- Community: outpatient management

The supplemental model uses provincial TB-specialized hospitals and TB-designated hospitals for:

- Hospitalization: treatment for severe TB, chronic TB and XDR-TB

TB hospitals serve as clinical centres to provide clinical training, laboratory support and technical assistance.

With support from partners, the next steps for finalizing the plan for PMDT are:

- To implement current projects and gain knowledge
- To further consult and revise the current tentative plan
- To fully integrate the plan into the next 10-year NTP plan
- For the State Council to authorize the plan.

The policy on MDR-TB control has been established within the NTP. The summary is shown in Table 20.

**Table 20.** Summary of NTP policy on MDR-TB treatment

| Items | Policy |
|---|---|
| Case finding strategy | Failure to Cat I and II, RAD, Relapse, Other retreatment, Contact with a known MDR-TB case, and nonconverter of smear after 2–3 months of start of treatment |
| Source of referral | Public facilities (incl.: DOTS clinics, HCs, and hospitals at national, provincial and district levels) |
| Treatment strategy | Both standardized (6ZKmLfxPasPto - 18ZLfxPASPto) and individualized |
| Method of provision of treatment | Partially hospitalized (two months ) and ambulatory DOT |
| Type of treatment supervisor | Home care DOT conducted by HCWs |

Cat = category; RAD = return after default; HCs = health centres; DOT = direct observed treatment; HCWs = health care workers; incl. = including; Z = pyrazinamid; Km = kanamicin; Lfx = levofloxacin; Pas = para-aminosalicylic acid; Pto = protionamide

## 4.3 The Lao People's Democratic Republic

The Lao People's Democratic Republic is the only landlocked country in South-East Asia, bordered by Cambodia, China, Myanmar, Thailand and Viet Nam. Its population was estimated at about 6 million in July 2004, dispersed unevenly across the country. Most people live in valleys of the Mekong River and its tributaries. Vientiane Prefecture, which includes Vientiane, the capital and largest city in the country, had about 600 000 residents. The country's population density is 23.4 per square kilometre. The median age of the population is 20, with the proportion of those under 15 years old at 39% in 2006. The population sex ratio (males per 100 females) was 99.2 in 2005. About 21% of the population lived in urban areas in 2006.

The mountainous geography and the low population density in many areas pose challenges to TB control activities in the Lao People's Democratic Republic, increasing difficulty in communication, monitoring and distribution of supplies and equipment. Staff in remote provinces and districts often receive limited support and have fewer resources for TB diagnosis, resulting in a high turnover of personnel. TB cases in distant villages have limited access to the district hospital due to distance and costs of transportation. Increased involvement of the private sector in TB control activities is expected due to economic progress in Vientiane and large provincial capitals.

**Figure 27.** The Lao People's Democratic Republic

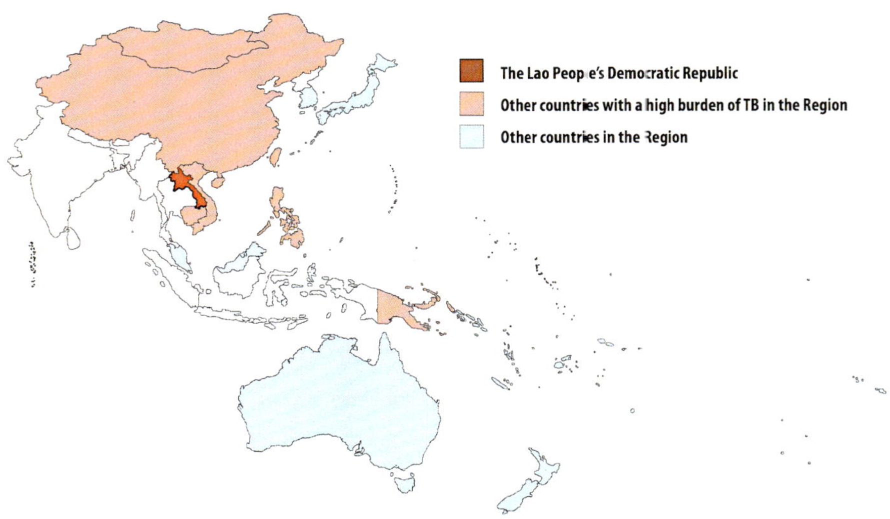


**Table 21.** Key indicators of TB control in the country, the Lao People's Democratic Republic, 2008

| | |
|---|---|
| Population (thousands) | 6205 |
| TB burden (2008 estimate) | |
| Incidence (all forms/100 000 population) | 150 [120–180] |
| Incidence (ss+/100 000 population) | 74 [59–89] |
| Prevalence (all forms/100 000 population) | 260 [170–400] |
| Mortality (deaths/100 000 population) | 32 [13–61] |
| Prevalence of HIV in adult incident TB cases (%) | 2 [1.8–2.4] |
| New multidrug-resistant TB cases (%)* | - |
| Previously treated multidrug-resistant TB cases (%)* | - |

- = data unavailable

**Table 22.** DOTS implementation, the Lao People's Democratic Republic, 2008

| | |
|---|---|
| Number of notified cases (new and relapse) | 4048 |
| Notification rate (new and relapse/100 000 population) | 65 |
| Notification rate (new ss+/100 000 population) | 50 |
| Case detection (new and relapse, %) Best [Low-High- estimates] | 44 [36–55] |
| Treatment success (2007 cohort new ss+, %) | 92 |

## Surveillance and epidemiology

Between 2000 and 2006, case notification rates increased significantly for all forms of TB from 42 to 69 per 100 000 population and for smear-positive TB from 29 to 53 per 100 000 population, respectively (Figure 28). However, both rates have remained stable between 2005 and 2008.

**Figure 28.** Trend of case notification rates (all forms of TB and smear-positive), the Lao People's Democratic Republic, 2000–2008

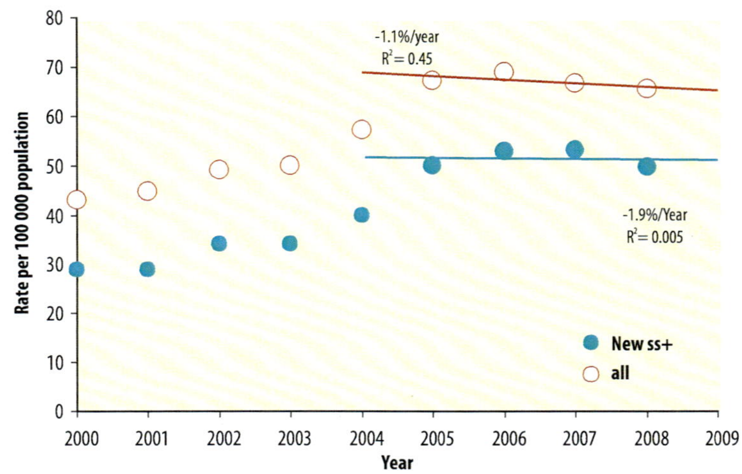


The notification rates for all forms of TB vary among provinces and are highest in Vientiane Municipality (108/100 000 population) and lowest in Xiengkhuang (11/100 000 population) (Figure 29). The provincial figures are available in Annex 8.

**Figure 29.** Geographical distribution of notification rates of all forms of TB, the Lao People's Democratic Republic, 2008

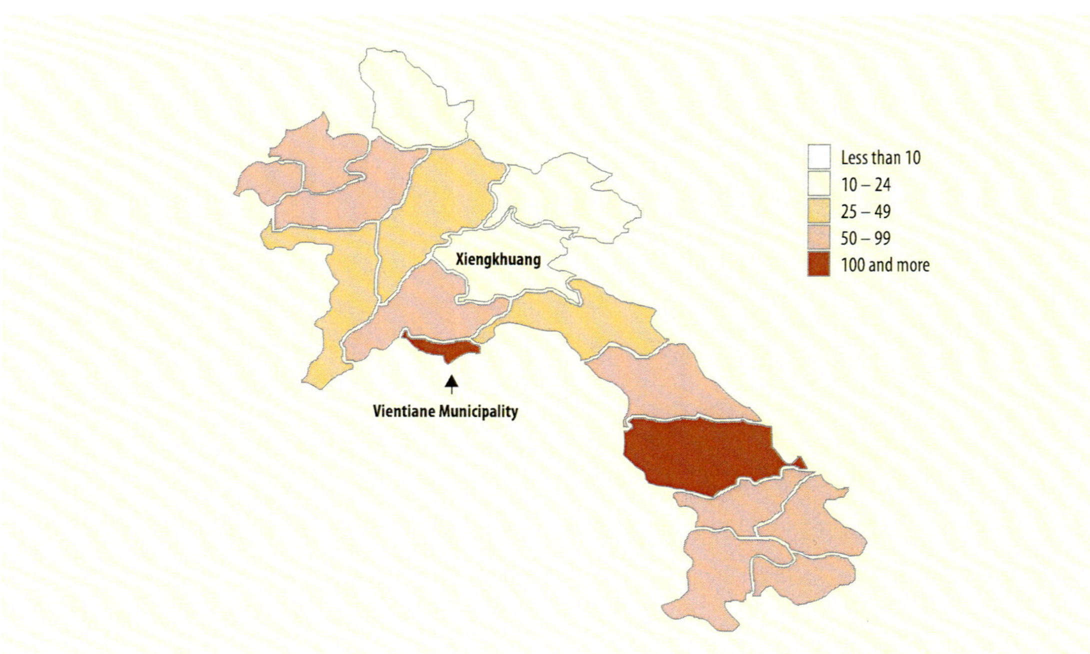

**Figure 30.** Distribution of forms of TB among new cases, the Lao People's Democratic Republic, 2003–2008

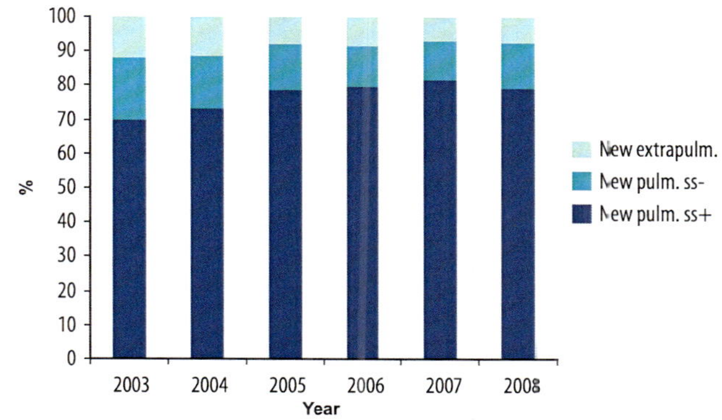


extrapulm. = extrapulmonary; pulm. = pulmonary; ss- or ss+ = sputum smear negative or positive

The distribution of forms of TB among new cases notified between 2003 and 2008 is shown in Figure 30. The proportion of smear-positive cases has increased from 70% in 2003 to 79% in 2008 while that of smear-negative and extrapulmonary cases have declined from 18% to 13% and from 12% to 8%, respectively.

**Figure 31.** Distribution of forms of TB among new and retreatment cases, the Lao People's Democratic Republic, 2003–2008

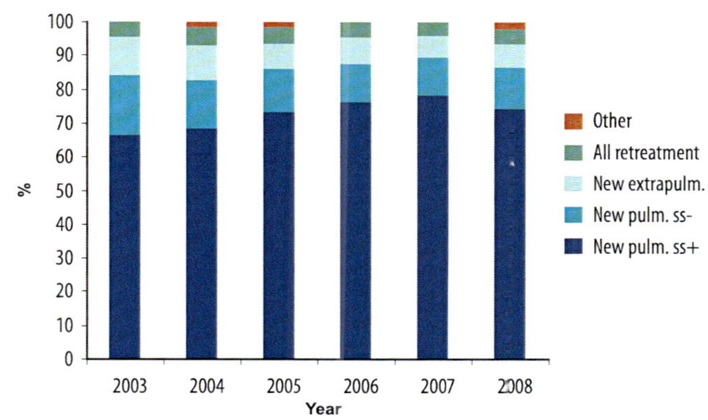


extrapulm. = extrapulmonary; pulm. = pulmonary; ss- or ss+ = sputum smear negative or positive

Since 2003, the proportion of the all retreatment cases among all notified cases has remained stable with a range between 2.5%–3.4% (Figure 31).

**Table 23.** Trend of DOTS performance indicators, the Lao People's Democratic Republic

| | 2000 | 2001 | 2002 | 2003 | 2004 | 2005 | 2006 | 2007 | 2008 |
|---|---|---|---|---|---|---|---|---|---|
| DOTS coverage (%) | 70 | 75 | 77 | 85 | 98 | 100 | 100 | 100 | - |
| Notification rate (new and relapse/100 000 population) | 43 | 45 | 49 | 50 | 57 | 67 | 69 | 67 | 65 |
| Notification rate (new ss+/100 000 population) | 29 | 29 | 34 | 34 | 40 | 50 | 53 | 53 | 50 |
| Case detection rate (new and relapse, %) | 25 | 27 | 30 | 31 | 35 | 42 | 43 | 42 | 44 |
| Treatment success (new ss+, %) | 77 | 76 | 75 | 79 | 86 | 90 | 92 | 92 | - |
| Retreatment success (ss+, %) | 61 | 52 | 66 | 54 | 78 | 87 | 82 | 86 | - |

The country has sustained high treatment success rates in both new smear-positive and retreatment cases between 2004 and 2007 (Table 23).

### MDR-TB activities

Lao People's Democratic Republic is establishing an MDR-TB treatment programme; a drug resistance survey (DRS) is planned for the first time; the National Reference Laboratory will be renovated to be biosafety level three (BSL-3) to be able to perform DST in 2010; and an additional two laboratories will provide culture services. An application to the GLC will be submitted to establish an MDR-TB unit. Funds already have been secured by Global Fund Round 7.

A policy on MDR-TB control has been established within the NTP. The summary is shown in Table 24.

**Table 24.** Summary of NTP policy on MDR-TB treatment

| Items | Policy |
|---|---|
| Case finding strategy | Failure to Cat I & II, RAD, Relapse, Other retreatment, Chronic TB cases, HIV-TB, contact with a known MDR-TB case |
| Source of referral | District and provincial referral hospitals |
| Treatment strategy | Standardized treatment (regimens to be defined) |
| Method of provision of treatment | Partially hospitalized (duration to be defined) |
| Type of treatment supervisor | HCWs |

Cat = category; RAD = return after default; HIV-TB = HIV-TB co-infection; DR-TB = drug resistant-TB; HCs = health centres; DOT = direct observed treatment; HCWs = health care workers

Table 25 summarizes the country's future plans related to MDR-TB treatment during the period 2009–2014. The NTP projected the number of MDR-TB cases based on an assumption that 1% of new and 10% of retreatment smear-positive cases would be incident MDR-TB cases, which gives about 50 cases per year.

**Table 25.** Future projections regarding MDR-TB treatment, the Lao People's Democratic Republic, 2009–2014

| End of | 2009 | 2010 | 2011 | 2012 | 2013 | 2014 |
|---|---|---|---|---|---|---|
| Number of culture facilities to be functional | 1 | 3 | 3 | 5 | 5 | 5 |
| Number of DST facilities to be functional | 0 | 1 | 1 | 1 | 1 | 1 |
| Number of MDR-TB treatment sites to be functional (including hospital- and health centre-based) | 0 | 1 | 1 | 3 | 3 | 3 |
| Number of cases to get DST for diagnosis for MDR-TB | 0 | 25* | 200 | 400 | 500 | 600 |
| Percentage of patients getting DST of total estimated number of smear-positive cases | 0 | 0.8% | 6.6% | 13% | 16% | 20% |
| Number of MDR-TB cases newly enrolled on treatment | 0 | 5 | 10 | 20 | 25 | 30 |
| Percentage of newly enrolled patients of total estimated number of MDR-TB cases | 0% | 10% | 20% | 40% | 50% | 60% |

* In 2010, only chronic cases (estimated to be about 25) will be tested for MDR-TB.

## 4.4 Mongolia

Mongolia is the fifth largest country in Asia with a size of 1.6 million sq km. It is landlocked between East and Central Asia and borders China and Russia. In 2007, the population reached 2.6 million, and the overall population density was 1.7 people per square kilometre, making it the least densely populated country in the world. The median age of the population is 25, with the proportion of those under 15 years old at 28.0% in 2006. The population sex ratio (males per 100 females) was 98.1 in 2005. About 57% of the population lives in urban areas: Ulaanbaatar, the capital and largest city, is home to about 38% of the population.

Major challenges in TB control activities in Mongolia include the vast distances between health facilities and communities and the poverty characterizing many TB cases. Most TB cases receive the first two months of treatment in hospital while the continuation phase is completed on an ambulatory basis. Prisoners, the homeless and the unemployed have been identified as vulnerable groups for TB; treatment success rates among these populations are lower compared with the general population. MDR-TB is a continuing challenge to TB control in Mongolia, especially among prisoners.

**Figure 32.** Mongolia

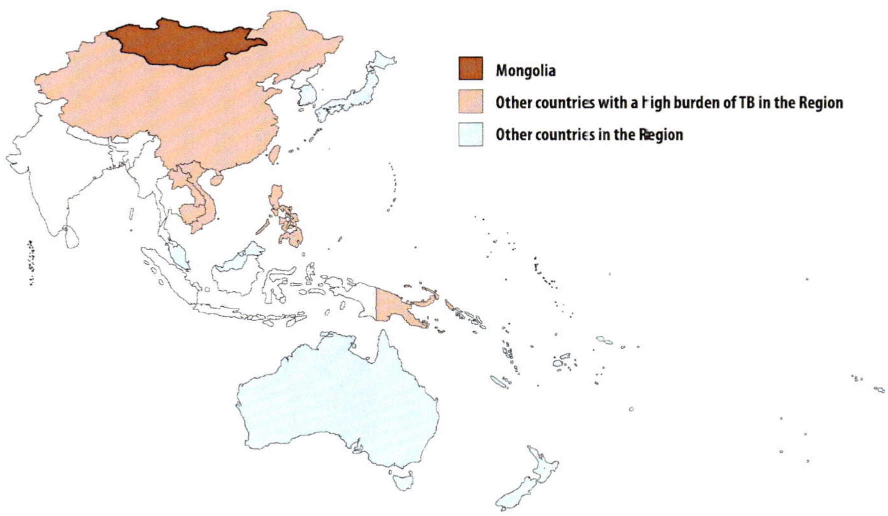


**Table 26.** Key indicators of TB control in the country, Mongolia, 2008

| | |
|---|---|
| Population (thousands) | 2641 |
| TB burden (2008 estimate) | |
| Incidence (all forms/100 000 population) | 210 [170–250] |
| Incidence (ss+/100 000 population) | 100 [84–120] |
| Prevalence (all forms/100 000 population) | 140 [29–280] |
| Mortality (deaths/100 000 population) | 21 [7.6–43] |
| Prevalence of HIV in adult incident TB cases (%) | 0.15 [0.12–0.18] |
| New multidrug-resistant TB cases (%)* | 1.4 |
| Previously treated multidrug-resistant TB cases (%)* | 27.5 |

*2008 Survey preliminary data

**Table 27.** DOTS implementation, Mongolia, 2008

| | |
|---|---|
| Number of notified cases (new and relapse) | 4490 |
| Notification rate (new and relapse/100 000 population) | 170 |
| Notification rate (new ss+/100 000 population) | 70 |
| Case detection (new and relapse, %) Best [Low-High estimates] | 83 [69–100] |
| Treatment success (2007 cohort new ss+, %) | 89 |

## Surveillance and epidemiology

Since 2000, case notification rates have increased for all forms and smear-positive TB cases from 126 to 194 per 100 000 population and 56 to 82 per 100 000 population in 2006, respectively (Figure 33). In 2008, the rates have decreased to 170 (all forms of TB) and 70 (smear-positive TB) per 100 000 population.

**Figure 33.** Trend of case notification rates (all forms of TB and smear-positive), Mongolia, 2000–2008

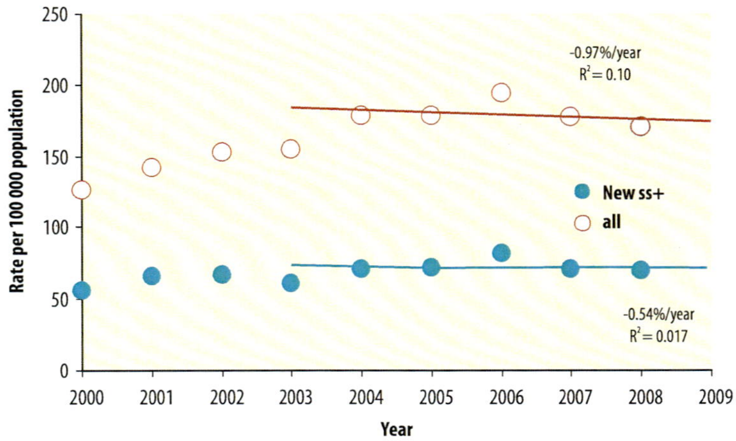


**Figure 34.** Geographical distribution of notification rates of all forms of TB, Mongolia, 2008

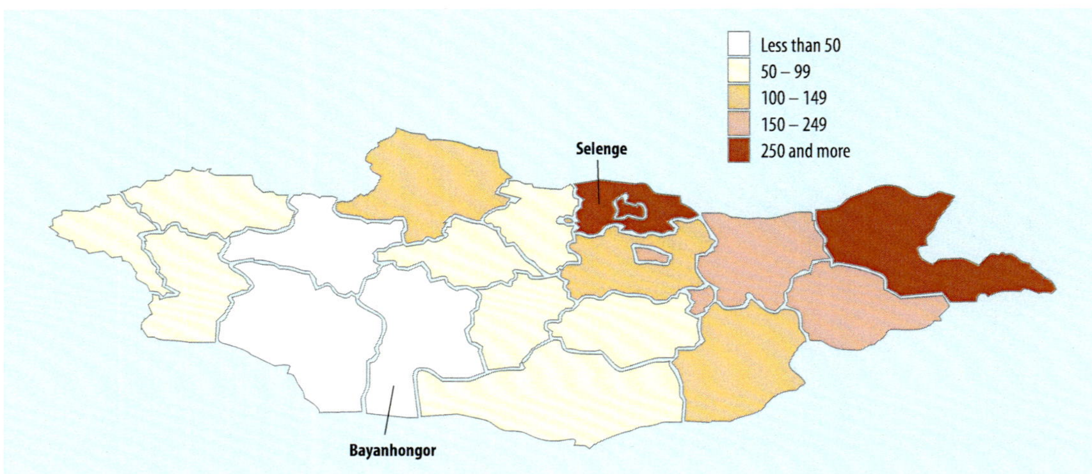


The notification rates for all forms of TB vary among provinces and are highest in Selenge (299/100 000 population) and lowest in Bayanhongor (28/100 000 population) (Figure 34). Provincial figures are available in Annex 8.

**Figure 35.** Distribution of forms of TB among new cases, Mongolia, 2003–2008

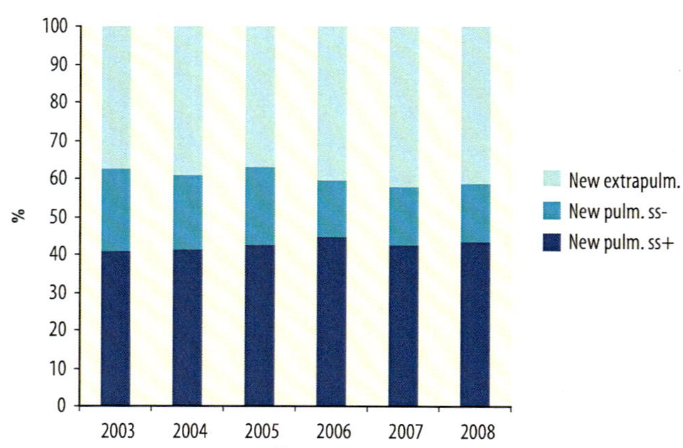


extrapulm. = extrapulmonary; pulm. = pulmonary; ss- or ss+ = sputum smear negative or positive

The distribution of forms of TB among new cases notified between 2003 and 2008 is shown in Figure 35. The proportion of smear-positive cases has remained stable with a range of 41% to 45%, while that of extrapulmonary cases varied between 37% and 42%. The proportion of smear-negative cases decreased from 22% to 15%.

**Table 28.** Trend of DOTS performance indicators, Mongolia, 2000–2008

| | 2000 | 2001 | 2002 | 2003 | 2004 | 2005 | 2006 | 2007 | 2008 |
|---|---|---|---|---|---|---|---|---|---|
| DOTS coverage (%) | 100 | 100 | 100 | 100 | 100 | 100 | 100 | 100 | - |
| Notification rate (new and relapse/100 000 population) | 126 | 142 | 153 | 155 | 178 | 178 | 194 | 177 | 170 |
| Notification rate (new ss+/100 000 population) | 56 | 66 | 67 | 61 | 71 | 72 | 82 | 71 | 70 |
| Case detection rate (new and relapse, %) | 63 | 71 | 76 | 77 | 88 | 88 | 95 | 87 | 83 |
| Treatment success (new ss+, %) | 87 | 87 | 87 | 87 | 88 | 88 | 88 | 89 | - |
| Retreatment success (ss+, %) | 71 | 72 | 69 | 72 | 70 | 73 | 68 | 76 | - |

The country has sustained high case detection and treatment success rates in new smear-positive cases between 2001 and 2008 (Table 28).

### MDR-TB activities

In 2006, the GLC approved the application submitted by the Ministry of Health to undertake a project of management of 375 MDR-TB patients. MDR-TB treatment started in June 2006 at the TB hospital with a 30-bed TB ward in Ulaanbaatar, where MDR-TB patients are hospitalized for a six-month intensive phase regardless of the clinical status. The prison TB hospital has 10 beds for MDR-TB, in which prisoners with MDR-TB are hospitalized for both the intensive and the continuation phase during their incarceration. The National Centre for Communicable Disease (NCCD) has a daily treatment unit for MDR-TB patients, where patients in the continuation phase receive ambulatory treatment with free lunch. In 2008, 65 MDR-TB cases were put on treatment. The treatment success rate for the cohort registered between 2006 and September 2007 was 71%. To improve access to MDR-TB treatment, the NCCD is planning to add 30 TB beds at the TB hospital and to establish two more ambulatory MDR-TB treatment sites in 2010.

The policy on MDR-TB control has been established within the NTP. The summary is shown in Table 29. Table 30 summarizes the country's future plans related to MDR-TB treatment during the period 2009–2014.

**Table 29.** Summary of NTP policy on MDR-TB treatment, Mongolia

| Items | Policy |
|---|---|
| Case finding strategy | Failure to Cat I and II, RAD, Relapse, Other retreatment, HIV-TB |
| Source of referral | Public facilities (incl. HCs, hospitals at national, provincial, and district levels) and private general practitioners |
| Treatment strategy | Standard (6 ZKmOflEthCs 18ZOflEthCs) |
| Method of provision of treatment | Partly hospitalized for six months followed by ambulatory management |
| Type of treatment supervisor | HCWs at daily treatment centre |

Cat = category; RAD = return after default; HIV-TB = HIV-TB co-infection; DR-TB = drug resistant-TB; HCs = health centres; DOT = direct observed treatment; HCWs = health care workers; incl. = including; Z = pyrazinamid; Km = kanamicin; Ofl = ofloxacin; Eth = etonamide; CS = cycloserine

**Table 30.** Future projections regarding MDR-TB treatment in the country, Mongolia, 2009–2014

| End of | 2009 | 2010 | 2011 | 2012 | 2013 | 2014 |
|---|---|---|---|---|---|---|
| Number of culture facilities to be functional | 1 | 2 | 3 | 3 | 3 | 3 |
| Number of DST facilities to be functional | 1 | 1 | 1 | 1 | 1 | 1 |
| Number of MDR-TB treatment sites to be functional (including hospital- and health centre-based) | 5 | 7 | 14 | 14 | 14 | 14 |
| Number of cases to get DST for diagnosis for MDR-TB | 396 | 406 | 416 | 427 | 432 | 437 |
| Percentage of patients getting DST of total estimated number of smear-positive cases | 80 | 80 | 80 | 80 | 80 | 80 |
| Number of MDR-TB cases newly enrolled on treatment | 108 | 167 | 170 | 170 | 170 | 170 |
| Percentage of newly enrolled patients of total estimated number of MDR-TB cases | 86 | 100 | 100 | 100 | 100 | 100 |

## 4.5 Papua New Guinea

Papua New Guinea is the largest country in the Pacific, occupying the eastern half of the island of New Guinea and offshore islands. Land mass area is 461 691 sq km, with the mainland making up 85% and about 600 smaller islands constituting the remaining 15%. The capital is Port Moresby. The country presents a challenging environment for all health programmes with its rugged terrain, very low population density and limited human resources development. Its population was 6.6 million in 2008. The average population density is just 13 people per square kilometre. The median age of the population is 20, with the proportion of those under 15 years old at 40% in 2006. The population sex ratio (males per 100 females) was 103.5 in 2005. Only 13% of the population lived in urban areas in 2006.

Government and churches provide nearly 100% of health care services in Papua New Guinea. Churches alone operate 46% of the health facilities, particularly those that are located in the periphery, using funds provided by the national government. Major challenges in TB control in Papua New Guinea include the limited availability of resources and staff, affecting implementation of TB control activities. Because of low performance of TB control in the country in previous years, the incidence of MDR-TB is likely to be rising, as noted by anecdotal reports of the increased number of MDR-TB cases identified by Australian TB services across the Torres Strait.

**Figure 36.** Papua New Guinea

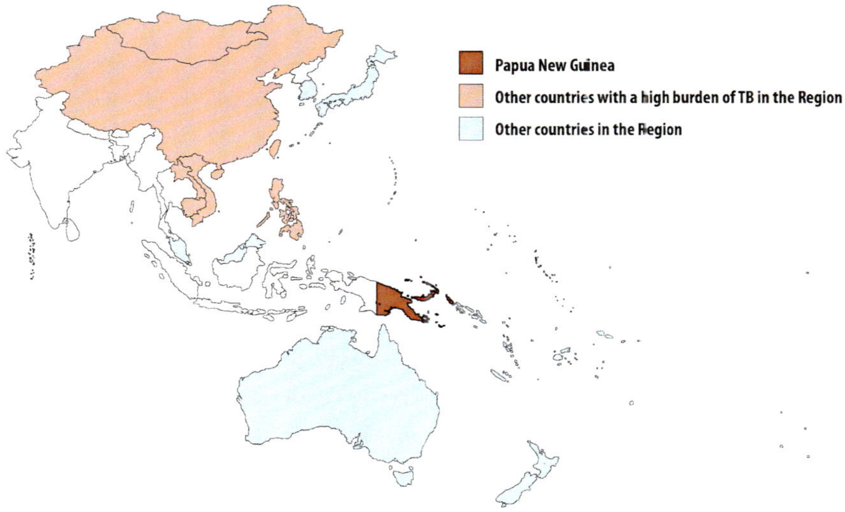


**Table 31.** Key indicators of TB control, Papua New Guinea, 2008

| | |
|---|---|
| Population (thousands) | 6577 |
| TB burden (2008 estimate) | |
| Incidence (all forms/100 000 population) | 250 [210–300] |
| Incidence (ss+/100 000 population) | 120 [110–150] |
| Prevalence (all forms/100 000 population) | 130 [37–290] |
| Mortality (deaths/100 000 population) | 21 [7.6–44] |
| Prevalence of HIV in adult incident TB cases (%) | 3.8 [3.0–4.6] |
| New multidrug-resistant TB cases (%)* | Not available |
| Previously treated multidrug-resistant TB cases (%)* | Not available |

**Table 32.** DOTS implementation, Papua New Guinea, 2008

| | |
|---|---|
| Number of notified cases (new and relapse) | 13 984 |
| Notification rate (new and relapse/100 000 population) | 213 |
| Notification rate (new ss+/100 000 population) | 35 |
| Case detection (new and relapse, %) Best [Low-High- estimates] | 85 [71–100) |
| Treatment success (2007 cohort new ss+, %) | 39 |

## Surveillance and epidemiology

Since 2000, case notification rates for all forms and for smear-positive TB cases have fluctuated with a range of 195 to 237 per 100 000 population and 24 to 40 per 100 000 population, respectively (Figure 37).

**Figure 37.** Trend of case notification rates (all forms of TB and smear-positive), Papua New Guinea, 2000–2008

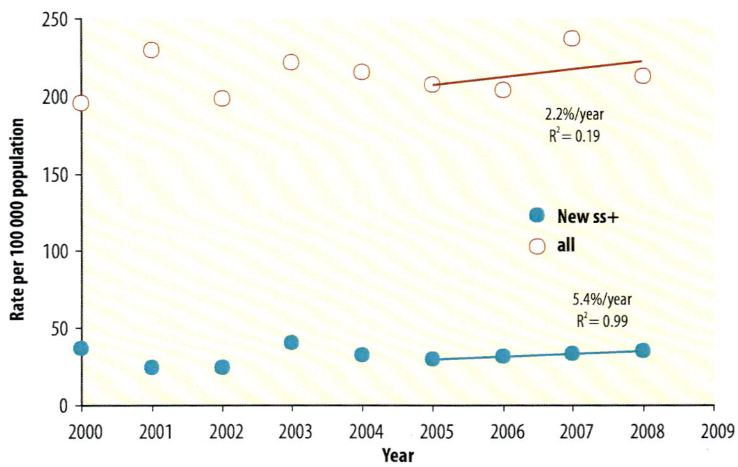


**Figure 38.** Geographical distribution of notification rates of all forms of TB, Papua New Guinea, 2008

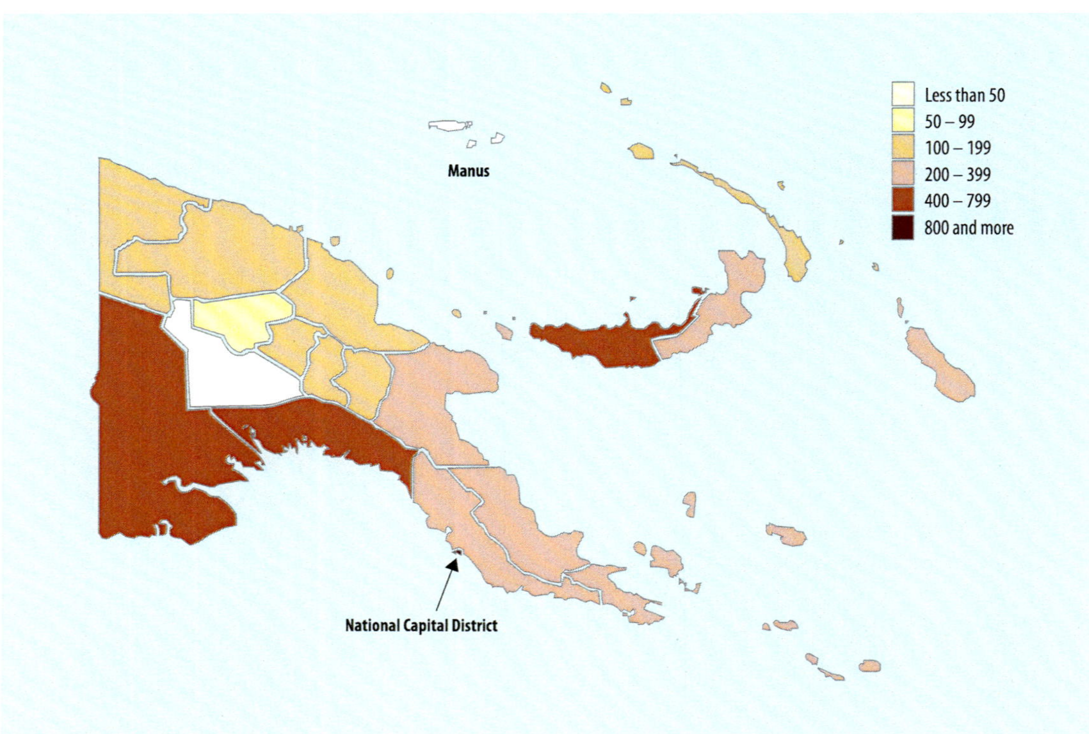

The notification rates for all forms of TB vary among provinces and are highest in the National Capital District (1131 per 100 000 population) and lowest in Manus (34 per 100 000 population) (Figure 38). Provincial figures are available in Annex 8.

**Figure 39.** Distribution of forms of TB among new cases, Papua New Guinea, 2003–2007

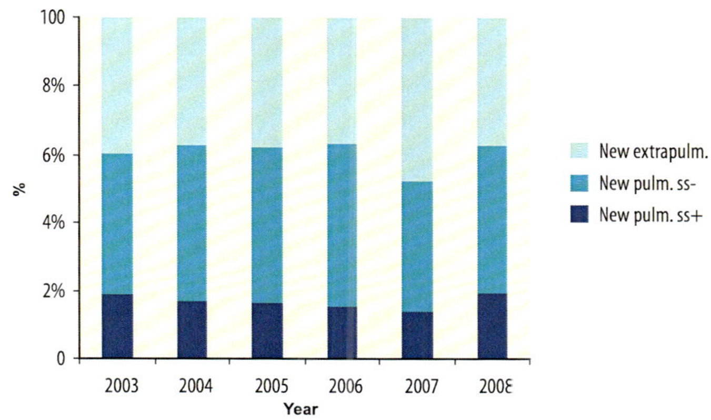


extrapulm. = extrapulmonary; pulm. = pulmonary; ss- or ss+ = sputum smear negative or positive

The distribution of forms of TB among new cases notified between 2003 and 2008 is shown in Figure 39. The proportion of smear-positive cases has fluctuated with a range of 14% to 19%, which are much lower than expected (about half of new cases). The proportions of smear-negative and extrapulmonary cases have also been fluctuating with a range of 38% to 48% and 37% to 48%, respectively.

**Figure 40.** Distribution of forms of TB among new and retreatment cases, Papua New Guinea, 2003–2008

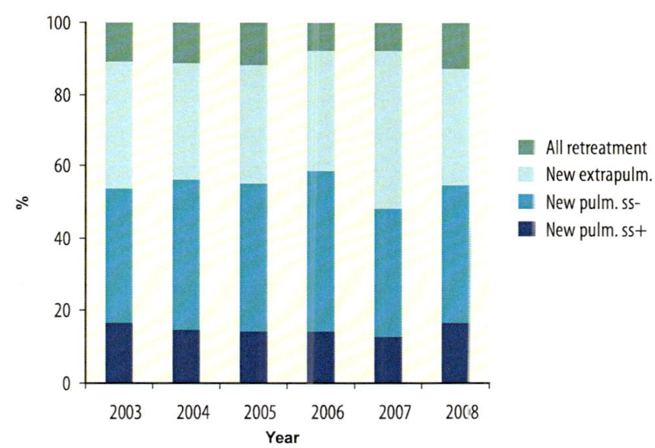


extrapulm. = extrapulmonary; pulm. = pulmonary; ss- or ss+ = sputum smear negative or positive

Since 2003, the proportion of all retreatment cases combined among new and retreatment cases has been fluctuating with a range of 6% to 10% (Figure 40).

**Table 33.** Trend of DOTS performance indicators, Papua New Guinea, 2000–2008

| | 2000 | 2001 | 2002 | 2003 | 2004 | 2005 | 2006 | 2007 | 2008 |
|---|---|---|---|---|---|---|---|---|---|
| DOTS coverage (%) | 8 | 13 | 24 | 46 | 47 | 53 | 40 | 14 | - |
| Notification rate (new and relapse/100 000 population) | 195 | 229 | 198 | 221 | 215 | 207 | 203 | 237 | 213 |
| Notification rate (new ss+/100 000 population) | 36 | 24 | 24 | 40 | 32 | 30 | 31 | 33 | 35 |
| Case detection rate (new and relapse, %) | 78 | 92 | 79 | 88 | 86 | 82 | 81 | 94 | 85 |
| Treatment success (new ss+, %) | 63 | 67 | 53 | 58 | 65 | 71 | 73 | 39 | - |
| Retreatment success (ss+, %) | 65 | 60 | 51 | 47 | 53 | 55 | n/a | n/a | - |

n/a = data unavailable

Treatment success urgently needs to be improved to be able to reduce the burden of TB in the country. (Table 33)

### MDR-TB activities

Pending the construction of a BSL-3 infrastructure in the laboratory and the delayed establishment of DST capacity at the Central Public Health Laboratory (CPHL), the country has not been conducting a diagnosis of MDR-TB according to the guidelines by using laboratory methods. As an interim measure, the CPHL plans to conduct culture for *Mycobacterium tuberculosis* from TB patients in the National Capital District and sending those with positive growth to the Queensland Mycobacterium Reference Laboratory (QMRL, Brisbane, Australia) to conduct further tests (DST). The CPHL will be upgraded to BSL-3 in early 2010 to be able to conduct DST in its own laboratory.

Also, the DRS initially planned between 2007 and 2008 with Global Fund support has now been delayed to start at the end of 2010. QMRL as the designated Supranational Reference Laboratory is planning to start a DRS in the Western province in mid 2010 with support from the Australian Agency for International Development (AusAID).

Various documents, such as an MDR-TB treatment guideline, an infection control operational guideline and an MDR-TB operational manual were being prepared or finalized. The policy on MDR-TB control is being drafted, and the summary is shown in Table 34. Table 35 summarizes the country's future plans related to MDR-TB treatment during the period 2009–2014.

**Table 34.** Summary of NTP policy on MDR-TB treatment, Papua New Guinea

| Items | Policy |
|---|---|
| Case finding strategy | Cat II failure |
| Source of referral | DOTS clinics, HCs |
| Treatment strategy | Standard (6CpEthOflCs 18EthOflCs) |
| Method of provision of treatment | Partly hospitalization for intensive phase and ambulatory treatment for rest of the treatment |
| Type of treatment supervisor | DOT watchers |

Cat = category; RAD = return after default; HIV-TB = HIV-TB co-infection; DR-TB = drug resistant-TB; HCs = health centres; DOT = direct observed treatment; HCWs = health care workers; Cp = capreomycin; Ofl = ofloxacin; Eth = etionamide; Cs = cycloserine

**Table 35.** Future projections regarding MDR-TB treatment in the country, Papua New Guinea, 2009–2014

| End of | 2009 | 2010 | 2011 | 2012 | 2013 | 2014 |
|---|---|---|---|---|---|---|
| Number of culture facilities to be functional | | 1 | 1 | 2 | 2 | 2 |
| Number of DST facilities to be functional | | 1 | 1 | 1 | 1 | 1 |
| Number of MDR-TB treatment sites to be functional (including hospital- and health centre-based) | | 7 | 15 | 19 | 19 | 19 |
| Number of cases to get DST for diagnosis for MDR-TB | | 50 | 200 | 300 | 400 | 400 |
| Percentage of patients getting DST of total estimated number of smear positive cases | | 1% | 3% | 4% | 6% | 6% |
| Number of MDR-TB cases newly enrolled on treatment | | 30 | 70 | 120 | 150 | 200 |
| Percentage of newly enrolled patients of total estimated number of MDR-TB cases | | 7% | 17% | 30% | 37% | 49% |

## 4.6 The Philippines

The Philippines is situated in the western Pacific Ocean and is categorized broadly into three main geographical divisions: Luzon, Visayas and Mindanao with more than 7000 smaller islands with a land area of 300 000 sq km. The population as of 2008 was about 90 million, giving a population density of 295 per square kilometre. The median age of the population is 22, with the proportion of those under 15 years old at 36% in 2006. The population sex ratio (males per 100 females) was 101.6 in 2005. About 63% of the population lived in urban areas in 2006.

The Philippines has built an effective infrastructure for TB control activities. Collaborative efforts between public and private sectors and the establishment of TB diagnostic committees successfully contributed to a dramatic increase in case detection and a decline in the number of over-diagnoses of smear-negative cases. Efforts were being made to build on the existing system to mainstream programmatic management of MDR-TB activities.

**Figure 41.** The Philippines

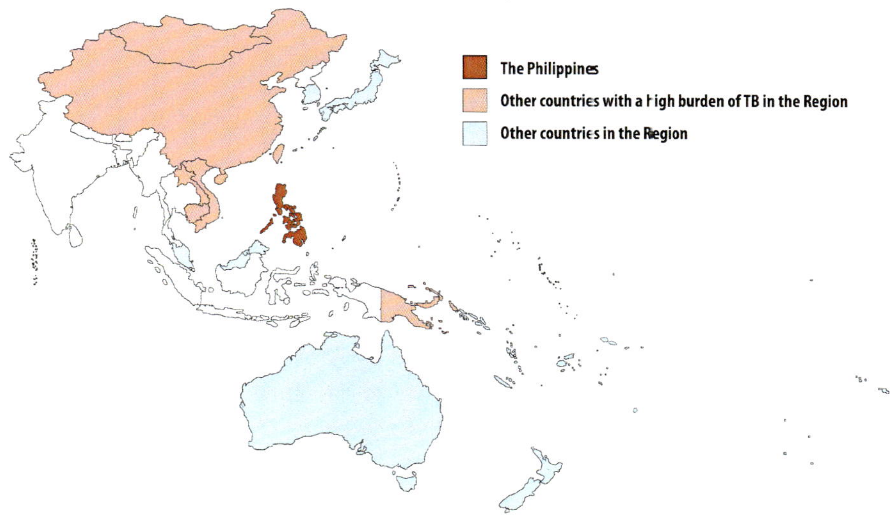


**Table 36.** Key indicators of TB control, the Philippines, 2008

| | |
|---|---|
| Population (thousands) | 90 348 |
| TB burden (2007 estimate) | |
| Incidence (all forms/100 000 population) | 280 [230–340] |
| Incidence (ss+/100 000 population) | 140 [110–170] |
| Prevalence (all forms/100 000 population) | 550 [500–600] |
| Mortality (deaths/100 000 population) | 52 [22–100] |
| Prevalence of HIV in adult incident TB cases (%) | 0.26 [0.19–0.34] |
| New multidrug-resistant TB cases (%)* | 4 |
| Previously treated multidrug-resistant TB cases (%)* | 21 |

*Surveyed in 2004.

**Table 37.** DOTS implementation, the Philippines, 2008

| | |
|---|---|
| Number of notified cases (new and relapse) | 139 603 |
| Notification rate (new and relapse/100 000 population) | 155 |
| Notification rate (new ss+/100 000 population) | 94 |
| Case detection (new and relapse, %) Best [Low-High estimates] | 54 [45–68] |
| Treatment success (2007 cohort new ss+, %) | 89 |

## Surveillance and epidemiology

Since 2000, the case notification rate for all forms of TB has fluctuated with a range of 139 to 171 per 100 000 population. After 2005, however, it started to decrease from 165 to 155 per 100 000 population with a rate of 2.6% per year (Figure 42). Likewise, the case notification rate for new smear-positive TB has fluctuated with a rage of 76 to 99 per 100 000 population and started to decrease since 2005 from 97 to 94 per 100 000 population with a rate of 1.1% per year.

**Figure 42.** Trend of case notification rates (all forms of TB and smear-positive), the Philippines, 2000–2008

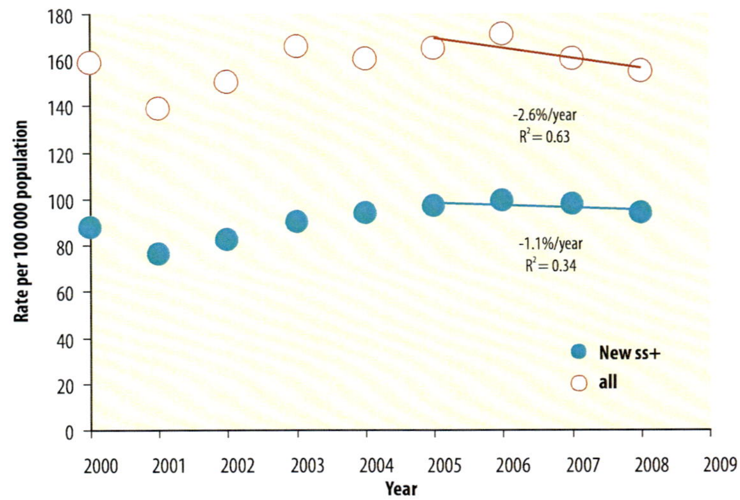


**Figure 43.** Geographical distribution of notification rates of all forms of TB, the Philippines, 2008

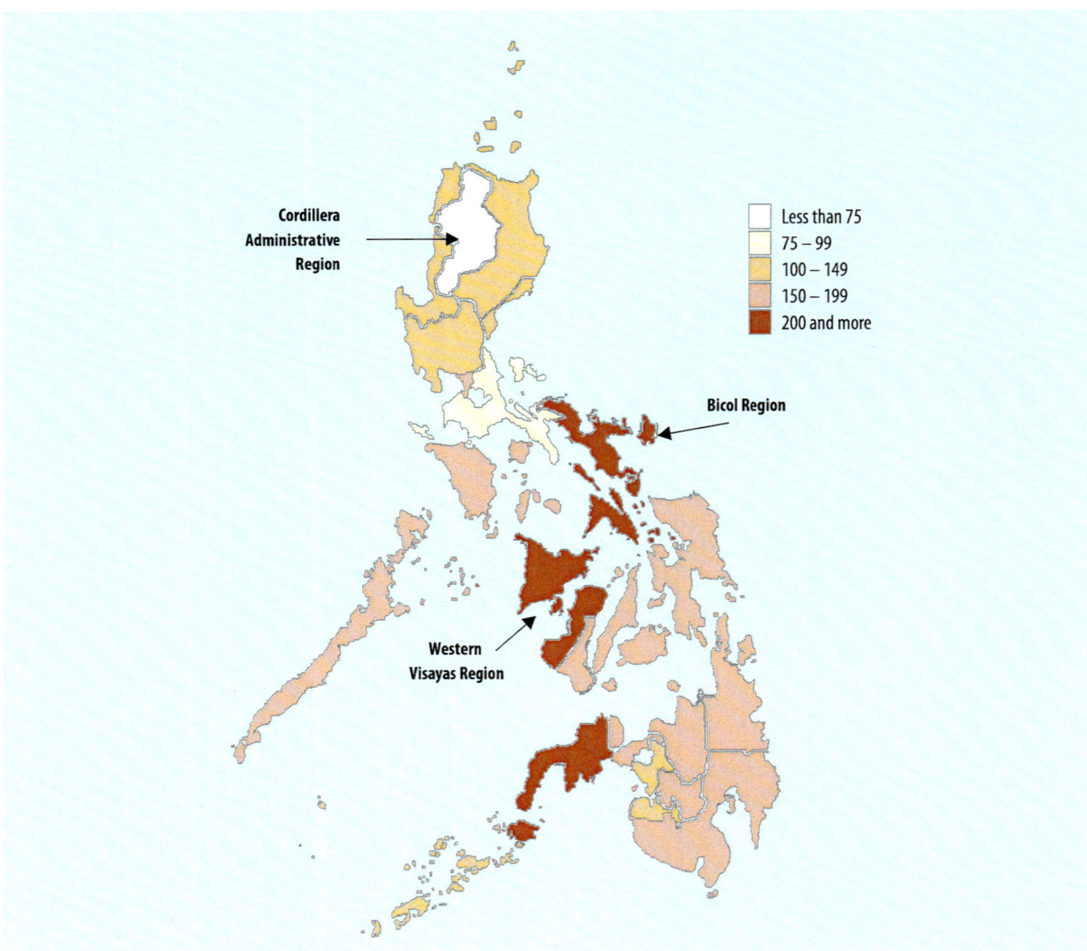

The notification rates of all forms of TB vary among regions in the Philippines and was highest in Bicol and the Western Visayas regions (250/100 000 population) and lowest in the Cordillera Administrative Region (74/100 000 population) (Figure 43). Regional figures are available in Annex 8.

**Figure 44.** Distribution of forms of TB among new cases, the Philippines, 2003–2008

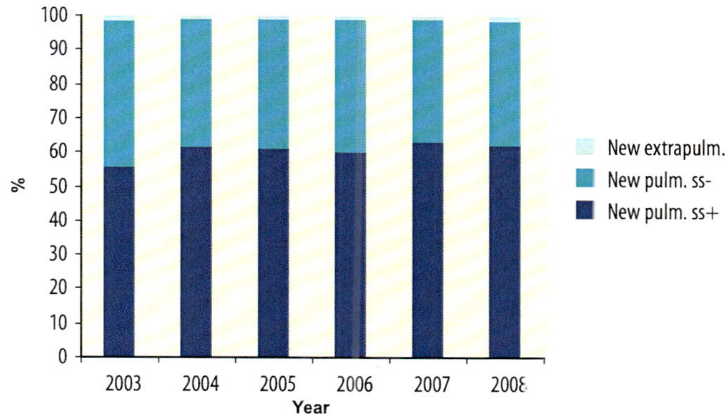


extrapulm. = extrapulmonary; pulm. = pulmonary; ss- or ss+ = sputum smear negative or positive

The distribution of forms of TB among new cases notified between 2003 and 2008 is shown in Figure 44. The proportion of smear-positive cases has slightly increased from 56% to 63%, while that of smear-negative cases has decreased from 43% to 36%. The proportion of extrapulmonary cases remained stable at under 1%.

**Table 38.** Trend of DOTS performance indicators, the Philippines, 2000–2008

| | 2000 | 2001 | 2002 | 2003 | 2004 | 2005 | 2006 | 2007 | 2008 |
|---|---|---|---|---|---|---|---|---|---|
| DOTS coverage (%) | 90 | 95 | 98 | 100 | 100 | 100 | 100 | 100 | - |
| Notification rate (new and relapse/100 000 population) | 158 | 139 | 150 | 166 | 160 | 165 | 171 | 160 | 155 |
| Notification rate (new ss+/100 000 population) | 88 | 76 | 82 | 90 | 94 | 97 | 99 | 98 | 94 |
| Case detection rate (new and relapse, %) | 47 | 42 | 46 | 52 | 51 | 53 | 57 | 55 | 54 |
| Treatment success (new ss+, %) | 88 | 88 | 88 | 88 | 87 | 89 | 88 | 89 | - |
| Retreatment success (ss+, %) | - | - | - | 76 | 53 | - | 76 | 72 | - |

The country has sustained a high treatment success rate in new smear-positive cases between 2000 and 2007 (Table 38).

### Policy on MDR-TB control and planned activities on MDR-TB

The Philippines had the first GLC-approved DOTS-Plus project in 2000. Since then, the project has expanded into the public sector and the community from initially having been limited to a private DOTS facility. In the past couple of years, it has been implemented as Programmatic Management of Drug Resistant-Tuberculosis (PMDT). By the end of 2009, 11 MDR-TB treatment sites for intensive phase, including six private facilities, and 194 sites for the continuation phase, including those for 13 faith-based organizations, NGOs and public-private mixed DOTS, have been established.

In terms of laboratory strengthening, five culture facilities, including three government and two NGO and private laboratories, are able to provide quality-assured culture tests. Of the five laboratories, three (the National TB Reference Laboratory, the Tropical Disease Foundation, Inc. and the Cebu TB Reference Laboratory) are also able to provide quality- assured DST to MDR-TB suspects.

Since 2000, more than 1500 MDR-TB cases have been enrolled for treatment. The treatment success rates for 2006 and 2007 cohorts were 59% (n = 134) and 63% (n = 314), respectively.

The NTP, in collaboration with its partners and local government units, plans to expand the PMDT nationwide with the goal of attaining 80% coverage of estimated MDR-TB cases and the target of detecting at least 15 000 MDR-TB patients and providing them with quality-assured MDR-TB treatment.

The policy on MDR-TB control has been established within NTP. The summary is shown in Table 39.

**Table 39.** Summary of NTP policy on MDR-TB treatment, the Philippines

| Items | Policy |
|---|---|
| Case finding strategy | Failure to Cat I and II, RAD, relapse, other, HIV-TB, non-converter of Cat II, contact of a DR-TB |
| Source of referral | Public facilities (inc. HCs, hospitals) and private facilities, and jails. |
| Treatment strategy | Individualized treatment based on DST results |
| Method of provision of treatment | Fully ambulatory DOT |
| Type of treatment supervisor | HCWs and volunteers at DOTS facilities |

Cat = category; RAD = return after default; HIV-TB = HIV-TB co-infection; DR-TB = drug resistant-TB; HCs = health centres; DOT = direct observed treatment; HCWs = health care workers

Table 40 summarizes the country's future plans related to MDR-TB treatment during the period 2009–2014.

**Table 40.** Future projections regarding MDR-TB treatment, the Philippines, 2009–2014

| End of | 2009 | 2010 | 2011 | 2012 | 2013 | 2014 |
|---|---|---|---|---|---|---|
| Number of culture facilities to be functional | 5 | 29 | 41 | 45 | 45 | 45 |
| Number of DST facilities to be functional | 3 | 5 | 5 | 5 | 5 | 5 |
| Number of MDR-TB treatment sites to be functional (including hospital- and health centre-based) | 11 | 32 | 42 | 42 | 42 | 42 |
| Number of cases to get DST for diagnosis for MDR-TB | 1728 | 2348 | 4474 | 4474 | 4474 | 4474 |
| Percentage of patients getting DST of total estimated number of smear positive cases | n/a | n/a | n/a | n/a | n/a | n/a |
| Number of MDR-TB cases newly enrolled on treatment | 864 | 1174 | 2237 | 2237 | 2237 | 2237 |
| Percentage of newly enrolled patients of total estimated number of MDR-TB cases | 21 | 45 | 61 | 65 | 80 | 75 |

## 4.7 Viet Nam

Viet Nam is located in the most eastern part of the Indochina Peninsula in South-East Asia. It is bordered by Cambodia, China and the Lao People's Democratic Republic. Its population is estimated to be 87 million people, being the 13th most populous country in the world. The population density is 252 people per square kilometre, with most people (73%) living in rural areas. The median age of the population is 25 years old. The population sex ratio (males per 100 females) was 96.8 in 2005.

Over the past a few years, Viet Nam has undergone a gradual change in its population structure. In 2006, the percentage of the population up to 14 years old was 26.4%, a decrease of 8.6% in comparison with 1999. However, the proportion of those over 64 years old increased rapidly (by 11%) over the same period.

Challenges faced by TB control activities in Viet Nam are related to the rapid spread of HIV since the early 1990s. The continuing spread of the HIV epidemic is expected to exacerbate the number of TB cases. However, a high political commitment at all levels supports national strategies to respond to the increasing number of TB-HIV cases. A TB control network with trained staff was established nationwide in the last decade. But access barriers to DOTS facilities remain in Viet Nam (e.g. distances, language and stigma). Vulnerable populations include the indigenous ethnic minorities, prisoners, people detained at drug rehabilitation centres, people living with HIV and IDUs.

**Figure 45.** Viet Nam

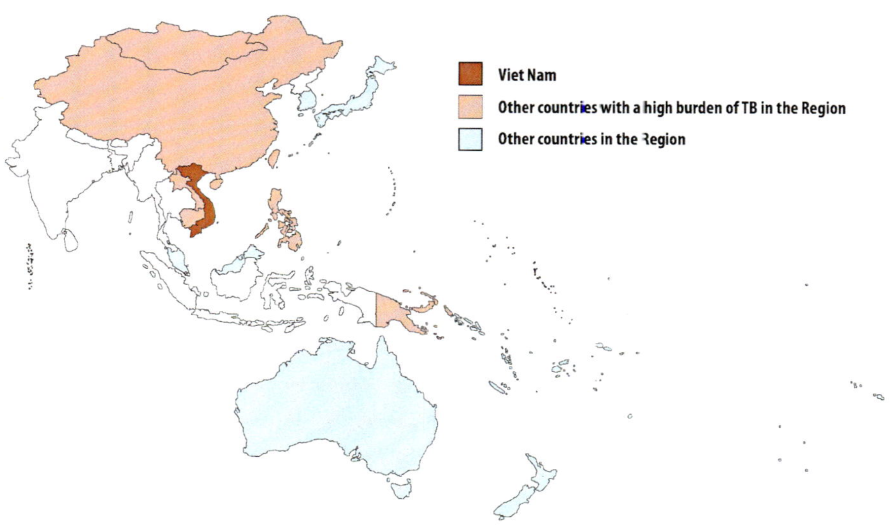


**Table 41.** Key indicators of TB control in the country, Viet Nam, 2008

| | |
|---|---|
| Population (thousands) | 87 096 |
| TB burden (2008 estimate) | |
| Incidence (all forms/100 000 population) | 200 [170–270] |
| Incidence (ss+/100 000 population) | 99 [82–140] |
| Prevalence (all forms/100 000 population) | 280 [140–480] |
| Mortality (deaths/100 000 population) | 34 [14–71] |
| Prevalence of HIV in adult incident TB cases (%) | 3.8 [3.0–4.5] |
| New multidrug-resistant TB cases (%)* | 2.7 |
| Previously treated multidrug-resistant TB cases (%)* | 19.3 |

*Surveyed in 2006.

**Table 42.** DOTS implementation, Viet Nam, 2008

| | |
|---|---|
| Number of notified cases (new and relapse) | 97 772 |
| Notification rate (new and relapse/100 000 population) | 112 |
| Notification rate (new ss+/100 000 population) | 61 |
| Case detection (new and relapse, %) Best [Low-High estimates] | 56 [41–68] |
| Treatment success (2007 cohort new ss+, %) | 92 |

## Surveillance and epidemiology

Since 2000, the case notification rate for all forms of TB has remained steady, ranging from 111 to 118 per 100 000 population (Figure 46). However, since 2002, the case notification rate for new smear-positive cases has decreased from 70 to 61 per 100 000 population at a rate of 2.4% per year.

**Figure 46.** Trend of case notification rates (all forms of TB and smear-positive), Viet Nam, 2000–2008

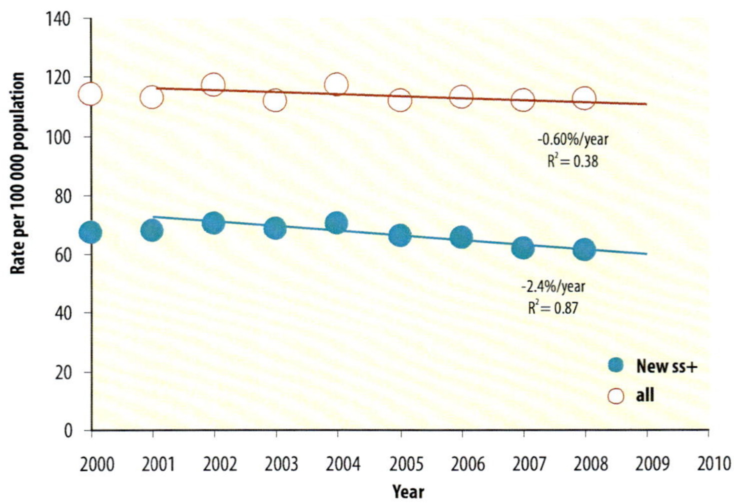


**Figure 47.** Geographical distribution of notification rates of all forms of TB, Viet Nam, 2008

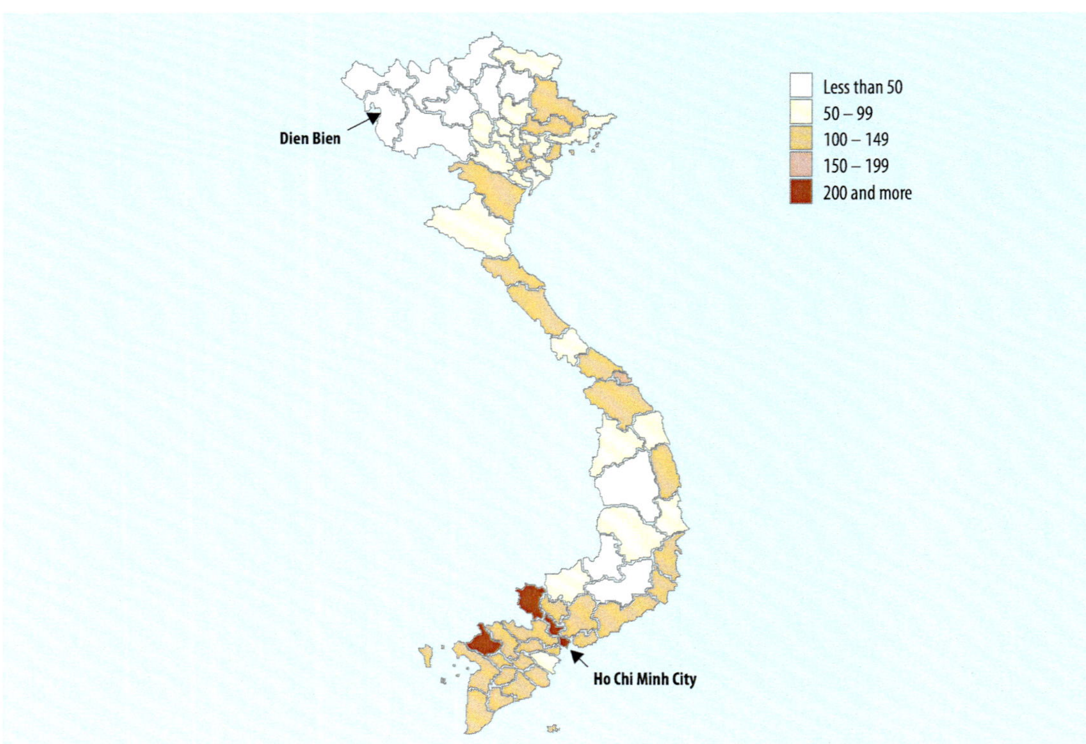

The notification rates of all forms of TB vary greatly among provinces in Viet Nam and are highest in Ho Chi Minh City (203/100 000 population) and lowest in Dien Bien (28/100 000 population) (Figure 47). Provincial figures are available in Annex 8.

**Figure 48.** Distribution of forms of TB among new cases, Viet Nam, 2003–2008

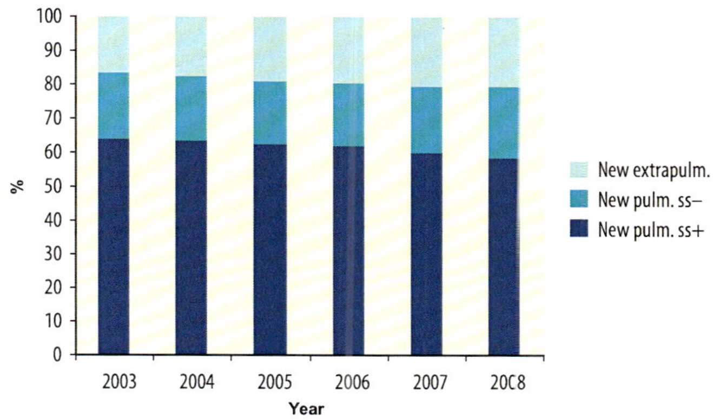


extrapulm. = extrapulmonary; pulm. = pulmonary; ss- or ss+ = sputum smear negative or positive

The distribution of forms of TB among new cases between 2003 and 2008 is shown in Figure 48. The proportion of smear-positive cases has decreased from 64% in 2003 to 59% in 2008, while that of extrapulmonary TB cases has increased from 17% in 2003 to 20% in 2008. The proportion of smear-negative TB has fluctuated with a range of 18% to 21%.

**Table 43.** Trend of DOTS performance indicators, Viet Nam, 2000–2008

| | 2000 | 2001 | 2002 | 2003 | 2004 | 2005 | 2006 | 2007 | 2008 |
|---|---|---|---|---|---|---|---|---|---|
| DOTS coverage (%) | 100 | 100 | 100 | 100 | 100 | 100 | 100 | 100 | - |
| Notification rate (new and relapse/100 000 population) | 114 | 113 | 117 | 112 | 117 | 112 | 113 | 111 | 112 |
| Notification rate (new ss+/100 000 population) | 67 | 68 | 70 | 68 | 70 | 66 | 65 | 62 | 61 |
| Case detection rate (new and relapse, %) | 56 | 56 | 56 | 56 | 56 | 56 | 56 | 56 | 56 |
| Treatment success (new ss+, %) | 92 | 93 | 92 | 92 | 93 | 92 | 92 | 92 | - |
| Retreatment success (ss+, %) | 79 | 85 | 85 | 85 | 84 | 83 | 78 | 82 | - |

The country has sustained high treatment success rates in new smear-positive cases between 2000 and 2007 (Table 43).

### Policy on MDR-TB control and planned activities on MDR-TB

Drug resistant-TB, including MDR-TB and resistance to isoniazid and streptomycin, has been one of the important challenges of the country. Viet Nam is estimated to produce about 4000 detectable new MDR-TB cases per year and is 13th among countries with a high burden of MDR-TB. The DRS conducted in 2006 revealed the countrywide MDR-TB prevalence to be 2.7% in new cases and 19% in retreatment cases. In addition, any isoniazid- and streptomycin-resistant cases were 19% and 23%, respectively, even among new cases caused by the extended use of streptomycin for Category I cases until 2007.

To respond to the problems related to drug resistant-TB, the NTP, supported by the Royal Netherlands Embassy and Global Fund Round 6, started PMDT implementation in May 2009 at Ho Chi Minh City TB Hospital by enrolling 100 MDR-TB patients. The NTP is scaling up the capacity against MDR-TB: building physical and technical laboratory capacity to perform quality-assured culture; DST and rapid molecular techniques for the diagnosis and follow-up treatment of MDR-TB cases; establishing physical, technical and human resource capacity to treat MDR-TB patients; carrying out education workshops on PMDT to engage all partners in support of MDR-TB treatment; and ensuring the uninterrupted supply of quality first- and second-line TB drugs to the MDR-TB treatment sites and other necessary supplies.

The NTP aims at treating up to 1500 (76% of estimated incidence cases) MDR-TB patients annually by 2015 and subsequently reducing the estimated incidence of smear-positive MDR-TB cases by 25% by 2015 compared with the estimated 2011 baseline. To assess the impact of MDR-TB control on prevalence, the NTP is planning to conduct another DRS in 2015.

The policy on MDR-TB control has been established within the NTP. The summary is shown in Table 44. Table 45 summarizes the country's future plans related to MDR-TB treatment during the period 2009–2014.

**Table 44.** Summary of NTP policy on MDR-TB treatment, Viet Nam

| Items | Policy |
|---|---|
| Case finding strategy | Failure to Cat I and II, RAD, relapse, other, contact of a MDR-TB |
| Source of referral | Provincial hospitals |
| Treatment strategy | Standardized treatment (6ZEKmLfxPtoCs[PAS], 12ZELfxPto Cs[PAS]) |
| Method of provision of treatment | Partly hospitalization for 1–2 months followed by ambulatory DOT |
| Type of treatment supervisor | HCWs and DOT watchers at home |

Cat = category; RAD = return after default; Z = pyrazinamide; E = ethambutol; Km = kanamycin; Lfx = levofloxacin; Pto = protianamid; Cs = cycloserine; PAS = para-aminosalicylic acid; DOT = direct observed treatment; HCWs = health care workers

**Table 45.** Future projections regarding MDR-TB treatment, Viet Nam, 2009–2014

| End of | 2009 | 2010 | 2011 | 2012 | 2013 | 2014 |
|---|---|---|---|---|---|---|
| Number of culture facilities to be functional | 2 | 17 | 17 | 17 | 20 | 25 |
| No. of DST facilities to be functional | 2 | 2 | 2 | 2 | 4 | 4 |
| Number of MDR-TB treatment sites to be functional (including hospital- and health centre-based) | 1 | 7 | 7 | 10 | 10 | 10 |
| Number of cases to get DST for diagnosis for MDR-TB | 300 | 1500 | 2730 | 2700 | 3300 | 3900 |
| Percentage of patients getting DST of total estimated number of smear positive cases | 0.5 | 2.2 | 3.9 | 3.6 | 4.2 | 4.8 |
| Number of MDR-TB cases newly enrolled on treatment | 100 | 500 | 910 | 900 | 1100 | 1300 |
| Percentage of newly enrolled patients of total estimated number of MDR-TB cases | 3.3 | 18 | 35 | 37 | 48 | 61 |

# 5 Summary of the TB epidemiologic indicators of Pacific island countries and area

**Figure 49.** Geographic distribution of the Pacific island countries and areas

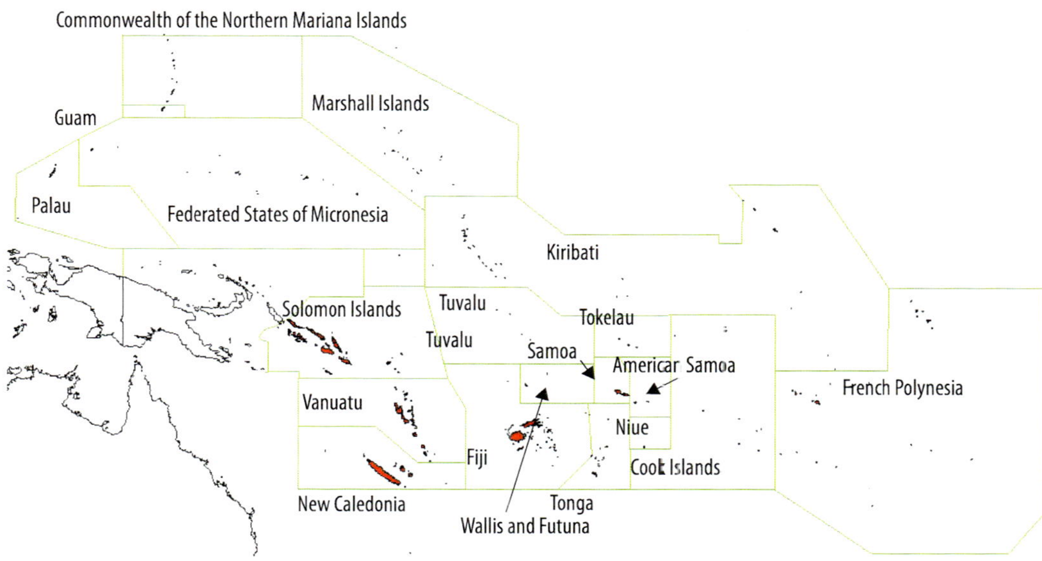


The boundaries shown and the designations used on this map do not imply the expression of any opinion whatsoever on the part of the World Health Organization concerning the legal status of any country, territory, city or area or of its authorities, or concerning the delimitation of its frontiers or boundaries.


The Pacific island countries and areas include American Samoa, Cook Islands, Fiji, French Polynesia, Guam, Kiribati, the Commonwealth of the Northern Mariana Islands, the Marshall Islands, the Federated States of Micronesia, Nauru, New Caledonia, Niue, Palau, Samoa, Solomon Islands, Tokelau, Tonga, Tuvalu, Vanuatu and Wallis and Futuna (Figure 49). Table 46 shows the key indicators of TB control in the Pacific island countries. Case notification rates for all forms of TB were highest in Kiribati (304/100 000 population) and lowest in Niue and Tokelau (0/100 000 population). Likewise, case notification rates for new smear-positive TB were highest in Kiribati (133/100 000 population) and lowest in American Samoa, Niue and Tokelau (0/100 000 population).

**Table 46.** Key indicators of TB control in the Pacific island countries and areas in the Region, 2008

| Country and area | Population (thousand) | Estimated incidence | | | | Treatment outcomes (%) | | | | |
|---|---|---|---|---|---|---|---|---|---|---|
| | | All forms | | ss+ | | | | | | |
| | | Number | Rate* | Number | Rate | cured | completed | died | failed | other |
| American Samoa | 67 | 3 | 5 | 0 | 0 | | | | | |
| Cook Islands | 20 | 2 | 10 | 2 | 10 | 0 | 100 | 0 | 0 | 0 |
| Fiji | 844 | 106 | 13 | 78 | 9 | 81 | 0 | 5 | 0 | 14 |
| French Polynesia | 266 | 50 | 19 | 20 | 8 | 85 | 0 | 12 | 0 | 4 |
| Guam | 176 | 89 | 51 | 31 | 18 | 89 | 0 | 6 | 0 | 6 |
| Kiribati | 110 | 335 | 304 | 147 | 133 | 79 | 14 | 7 | 0 | 0 |
| Marshall Islands | 61 | 125 | 206 | 28 | 46 | 93 | 4 | 0 | 0 | 4 |
| Federated States of Micronesia | 97 | 164 | 169 | 38 | 39 | 25 | 40 | 8 | 2 | 25 |
| Nauru | 10 | 5 | 50 | 2 | 20 | 0 | 100 | 0 | 0 | 0 |
| New Caledonia | 246 | 44 | 18 | 9 | 4 | 69 | 8 | 23 | 0 | 0 |
| Niue | 1 | 0 | 0 | 0 | 0 | | | | | |
| Commonwealth of the Northern Mariana Islands | 85 | 28 | 33 | 13 | 15 | 0 | 92 | 0 | 0 | 8 |
| Palau | 21 | - | - | - | - | - | - | - | - | - |
| Samoa | 179 | 12 | 7 | 6 | 3 | 85 | 8 | 0 | 8 | 0 |
| Solomon Islands | 511 | 387 | 76 | 140 | 27 | 75 | 17 | 6 | 0 | 2 |
| Tokelau | 1 | 0 | 0 | 0 | 0 | | | | | |
| Tonga | 104 | 13 | 13 | 11 | 11 | 93 | 0 | 7 | 0 | 0 |
| Tuvalu | 10 | 17 | 170 | 9 | 90 | 56 | 19 | 13 | 0 | 13 |
| Vanuatu | 234 | 103 | 44 | 45 | 19 | 81 | 12 | 2 | 0 | 5 |
| Wallis and Futuna | 15 | - | - | - | - | - | - | - | - | - |

Notification rates are per 100 000 population.
ss+ = smear-positive; - = data were not available;
The blanks in treatment outcomes in American Samoa, Niue, and Tokelau indicate no case was registered for new smear-positive category in 2007.

Trends of cases notification rates vary across the Pacific island countries (Figure 50). The fluctuation of rates over time can be attributed to its small population and/or the small number of cases that were reported.

**Figure 50.** Trends of case notification rates (all forms of TB and smear-positive cases) in the Pacific island countries and areas n the Region, 1993–2008[13]

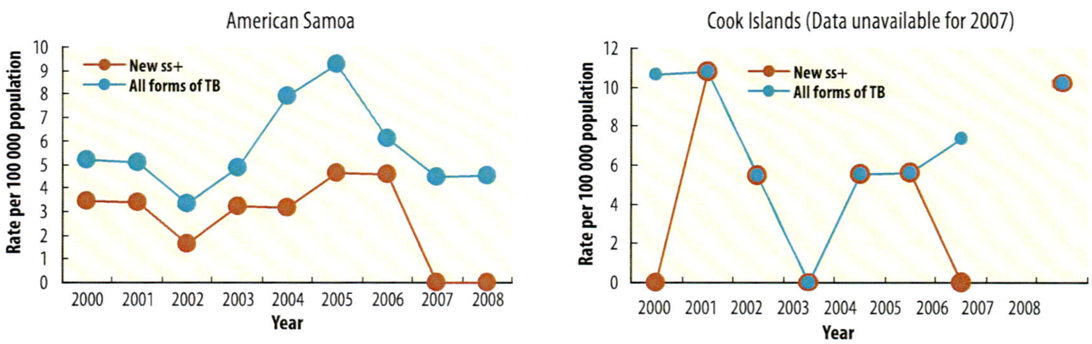


13 Tokelau is not shown here since no case was notified since 1995.

### Fiji

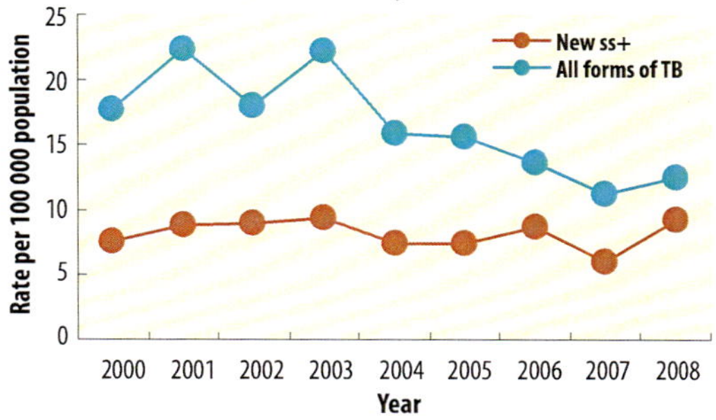


### French Polynesia

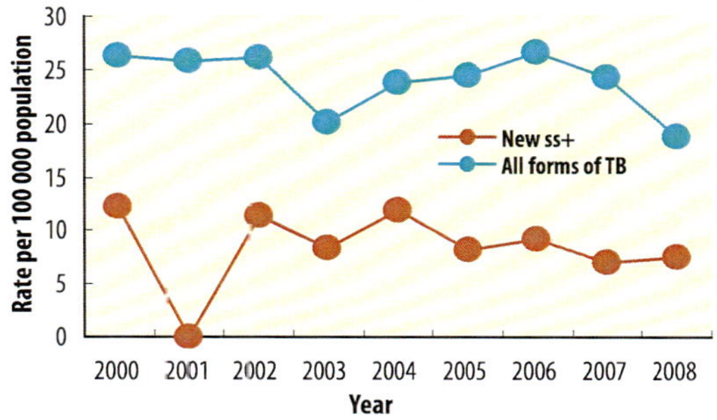


### Guam

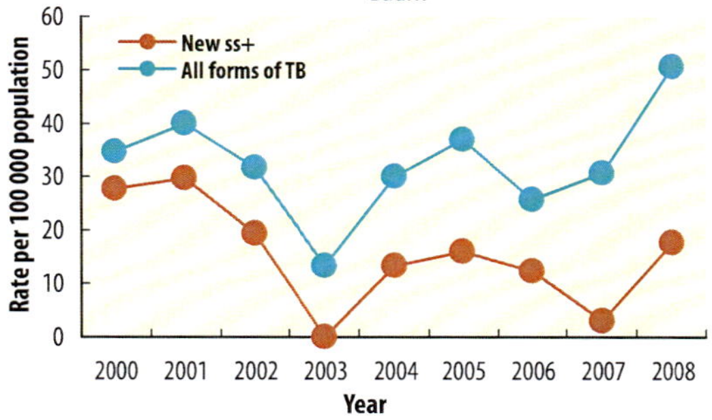


### Kiribati

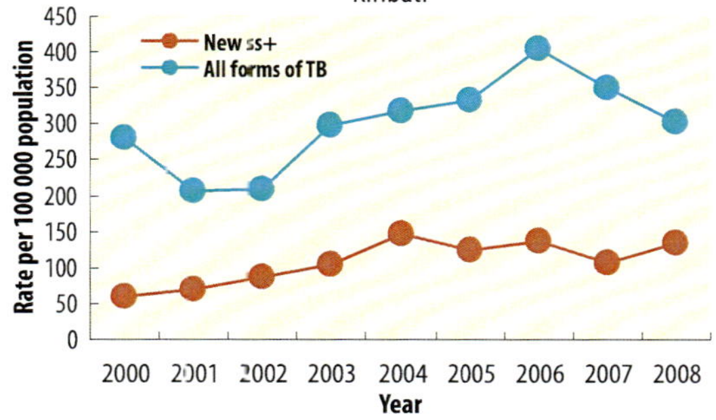


### Marshall Islands

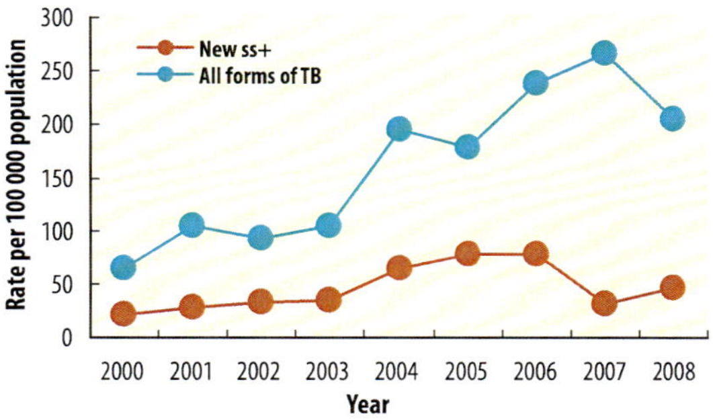


### Federated States of Micronesia

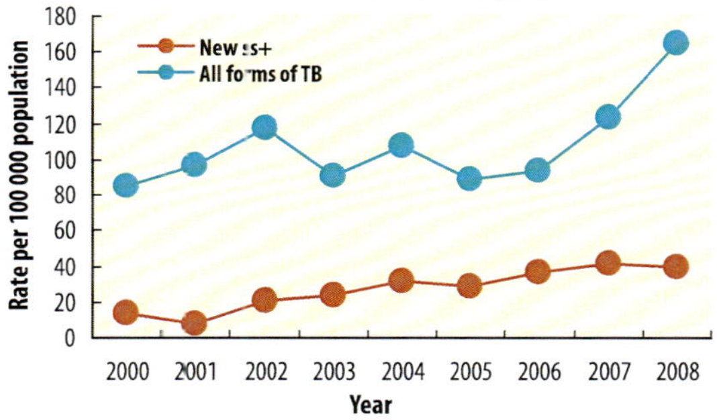


### Nauru (Data unavailable for 2004)

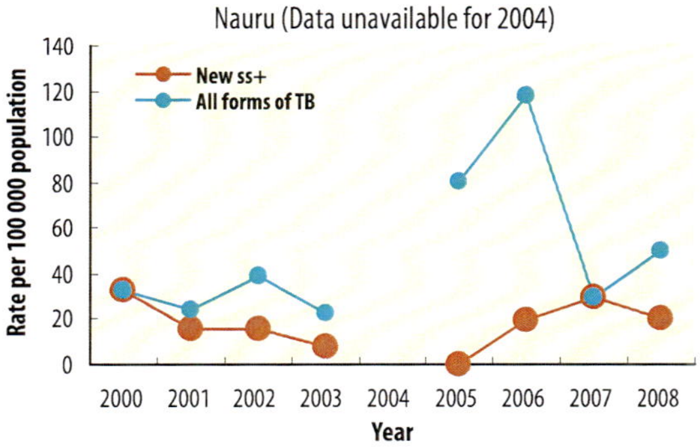


### New Caledonia

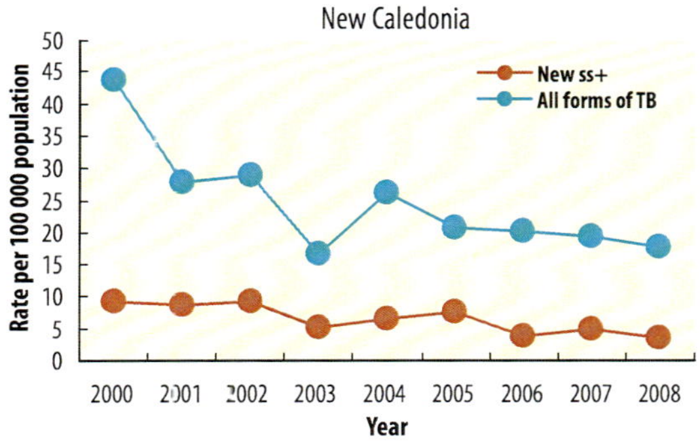


### Niue

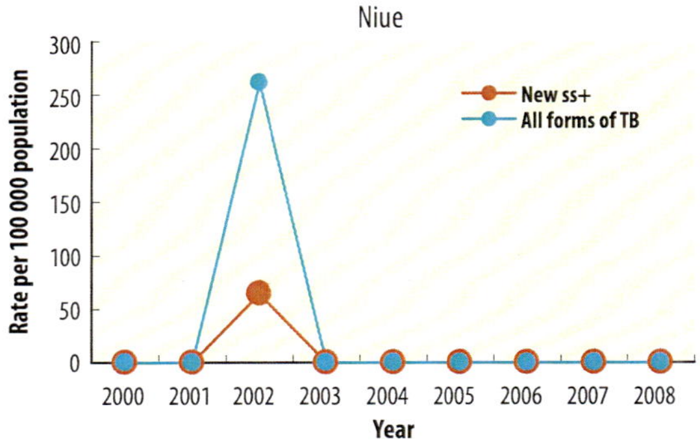


### Commonwealth of the Northern Mariana Islands

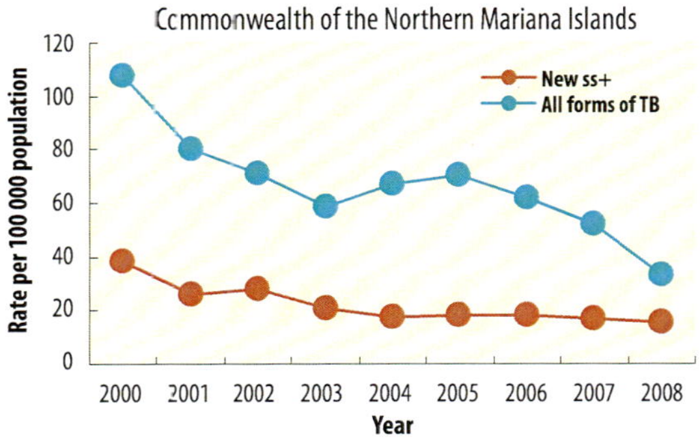

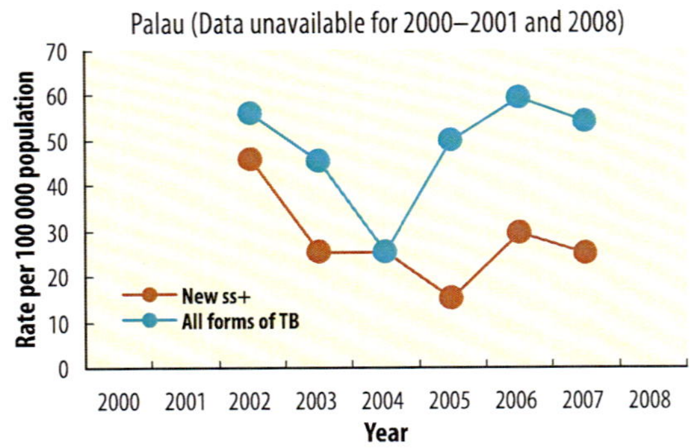
Palau (Data unavailable for 2000–2001 and 2008)
Rate per 100 000 population
Year
New ss+
All forms of TB

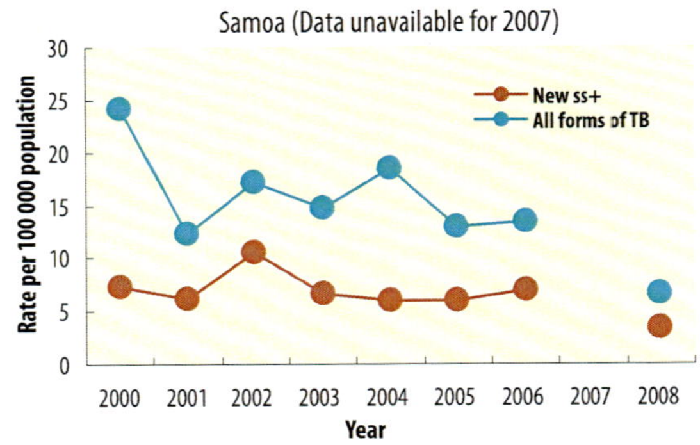
Samoa (Data unavailable for 2007)
Rate per 100 000 population
Year
New ss+
All forms of TB

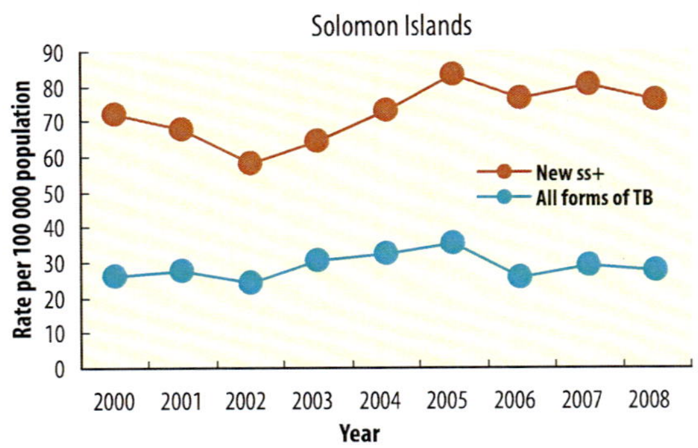
Solomon Islands
Rate per 100 000 population
Year
New ss+
All forms of TB

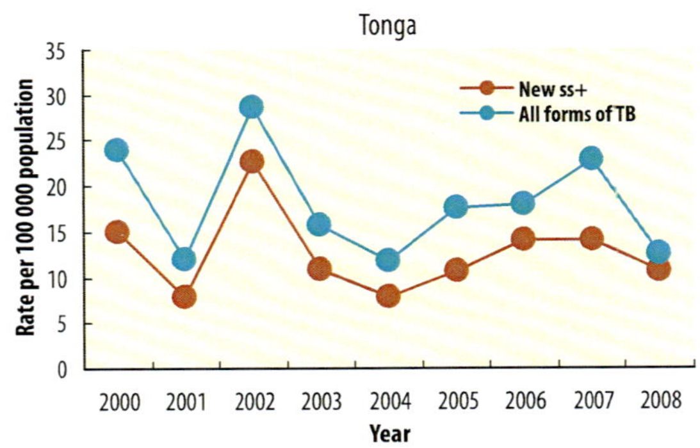
Tonga
Rate per 100 000 population
Year
New ss+
All forms of TB

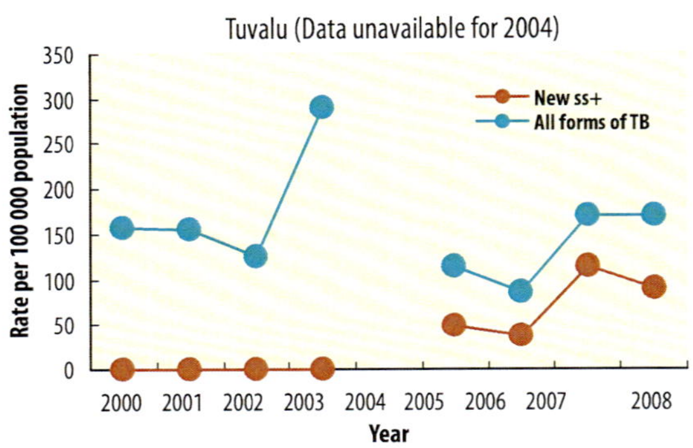
Tuvalu (Data unavailable for 2004)
Rate per 100 000 population
Year
New ss+
All forms of TB

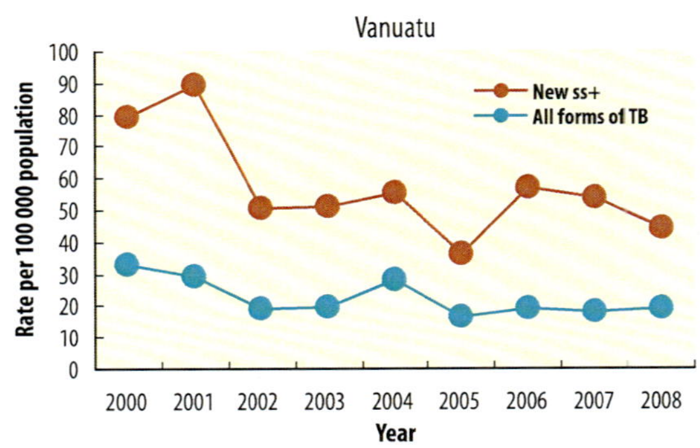
Vanuatu
Rate per 100 000 population
Year
New ss+
All forms of TB

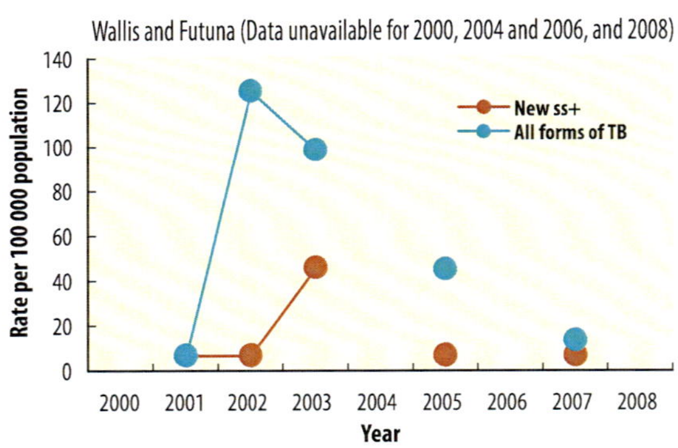
Wallis and Futuna (Data unavailable for 2000, 2004 and 2006, and 2008)
Rate per 100 000 population
Year
New ss+
All forms of TB

# Annexes

## Annex 1: Estimation of prevalence and TB mortality rates

Estimates and methodology used for this report are taken from 'Global Tuberculosis Control – a short update to the 2009 report" (WHO/HTM/TB/2009.426).

Concerning the most recent development of moving away from estimates of the case detection rate for sputum smear-positive pulmonary TB please refer to chapter 4.3 and Box 6 of "Global Tuberculosis Control 2010" (WHO/HTM/TB/2010.7).

## Annex 2: Estimation of MDR-TB prevalence

Based on drug resistance data reported from 114 countries and two special administrative regions of China, logistic regression models were fitted to estimate the proportion of MDR-TB among new, previously treated, and combined TB cases for a further 69 countries and areas for which surveyed data were not available. The estimated number of new TB cases by country and area was used to calculate the estimated number of MDR-TB cases that occurred among new cases. To estimate the number of previously treated cases for each country and area, the ratio of notified retreatment cases to notified new cases in 2008 was multiplied by the total number of new cases estimated to have occurred in the same year; therefore the total number of estimated case includes estimated retreatment cases.

## Annex 3: Definitions

### 1. Definitions of tuberculosis cases

**A case of tuberculosis:** A patient in whom tuberculosis (TB) has been bacteriologically confirmed or has been diagnosed by a clinician. Any person given treatment for TB should be recorded.

**All forms:** The sum of new smear-positive pulmonary, relapse, new smear-negative pulmonary and extrapulmonary cases.

**New smear-positive pulmonary TB:**[14] A patient who has never received treatment for TB, or who has taken anti-TB drugs for less than 30 days and who has one of the following:

- two or more initial sputum smear examinations positive for acid fast bacilli (AFB);
- one sputum examination positive for AFB plus radiographic abnormalities consistent with active pulmonary TB as determined by a clinician; or
- one sputum specimen positive for AFB and at least one sputum that is culture-positive for AFB.

**New smear-negative pulmonary tuberculosis:** A case of pulmonary TB that does not meet the above definition for smear-positive TB.

**Extrapulmonary tuberculosis:** TB of organs other than the lungs, e.g., pleura, lymph nodes, abdomen, genito-urinary tract, skin, joints, bones, meninges. Diagnosis should be based on one culture-positive specimen, or histological or strong clinical evidence consistent with active extrapulmonary TB, followed by a decision by a clinician to treat with a full course of anti-TB chemotherapy. (A patient diagnosed with both pulmonary and extrapulmonary TB should be classified as a case of pulmonary TB.)

---

14 The case definition of new smear-positive changed in 2007 and will be applied in future regional reports.

**Retreatment case:** Patient previously treated for TB, undergoing treatment for a new episode of bacteriologically positive (sputum smear or culture) TB.

**Relapse:** A patient previously treated for TB and declared cured or treatment completed, who is later diagnosed with bacteriologically positive (sputum smear or culture) TB.

## 2. Definitions of treatment outcome

| | |
|---|---|
| Cured | Former smear-positive patient who was smear-negative in the last month of treatment, and on at least one previous occasion. |
| Completed treatment | A patient who has completed treatment but who does not meet the criteria to be classified either as a cure or a failure. |
| Treatment success | The sum of patients who are cured and those who have completed treatment. |
| Died | A patient who dies for any reason during the course of treatment. |
| Failure | A smear-positive patient who remained smear-positive at five months or later during treatment. |
| Defaulted | A patient who has interrupted treatment for two consecutive months or more. |
| Transferred out | A patient who has been transferred to another recording and reporting unit and for whom the treatment outcome is not known. |
| Not evaluated | A patient who did not have the treatment outcome evaluated.<br>Note: In countries where culture is current practice, patients can be classified as cured or failed based on culture results. |

## 3. Indicators to assess treatment outcome

**Cure rate:** Proportion of cured cases out of all cases registered in a given period (2007, in this report).

**Treatment success rate:** The sum of the proportion of patients who were cured and patients who completed treatment out of all cases registered in a given period. The global target is a 85% cure rate and a greater treatment success rate.

The cure rate and the treatment success rate are expressed as a percentage of registered cases. The number of new cases registered for treatment in 2007 (reported in 2009) is compared to the number of cases notified as smear-positive in 2007 (reported in 2008). Differences may arise because NTPs do not compile data at the end of each calendar year, diagnoses may be incorrect, patients are lost between diagnosis and the start of treatment, or records may be lost. All registered cases should be evaluated. Data on the six standard, mutually exclusive outcomes of treatment are compiled. These figures are reported as percentages of all registered cases. When a country or territory states the number of patients registered for treatment, but gives no outcomes, no result is reported, rather than reporting zero treatment success. Although treatment outcomes are expressed as percentages, they are referred to as rates. The six possible outcomes plus the fraction of cases not evaluated add up to 100%. If the number of registered cases is lower than the sum of the six outcomes or is missing, the denominator for treatment success will be the number evaluated or the number of smear-positive cases notified in the previous year, whichever is greater.

## 4. Case detection rate and DOTS detection rate

### Directly observed treatment, short-course (DOTS)

The recommended strategy for TB control is comprised of:

- political commitment with increased and sustained financing;
- case detection through quality-assured bacteriology;
- standardized treatment with supervision and patient support;
- an effective drug supply and management system; and
- monitoring and evaluation system, and impact measurement.

### Targets for TB control established by the World Health Assembly (1991)

- To cure 85% of the sputum smear-positive TB cases detected.
- To detect 70% of the estimated new sputum smear-positive TB cases.

Case notifications represent only a fraction of the true number of cases in a country or territory because the effective coverage of the NTP may be incomplete.

The estimated cases detection rate for new smear positive TB cases is defined as:

$$\text{Case detection rate new smear positive TB cases (\%)} = \frac{\text{Annual new smear-positive notifications (country and territory)}}{\text{Estimated annual new smear-positive incidence (country and territory)}}$$

## 5. Definitions of MDR-TB and XDR-TB

| | |
|---|---|
| MDR-TB, or multidrug-resistant TB | Strains of TB that are resistant to at least the two main first-line anti-TB drugs—isoniazid and rifampicin. |
| XDR-TB, or extensively drug-resistant TB | TB that is resistant to any fluoroquinolone, and at least one of three injectable second-line drugs (capreomycin, kanamycin, and amikacin), in addition to MDR-TB. The WHO Global Task Force on XDR-TB agreed on this definition of XDR-TB in October 2006. |

# Annex 4: Formulas for estimating tuberculosis incidence, prevalence, and mortality

Estimates of the burden of TB (incidence, prevalence, and mortality) have been improved and updated following 18 months of work by an expert group convened by the WHO Global Task Force on TB Impact Measurement as well as increased availability of data. The number of countries with direct measurements of HIV infection in TB patients has risen to 103 (up from 64 in the 2008 round of data collection), and TB mortality is now based on direct measurements from vital registration systems for 89 countries (compared with three for which such direct measurements were used in previous reports). Estimates have also been updated using in-depth analyses and country consultations conducted during a series of regional workshops and country missions in 2009. All estimates are provided with uncertainty intervals; this will become routine practice in all future reports. The detailed methods used to produce estimates of the burden of TB can be available from in Annex of the update to the 2009 Global Report.[15] The estimates for countries and areas in the Region will be re-assessed in the coming years.

15 pp. 32–38 of Global tuberculosis control –a short update to the 2009 report (WHO/HTM/TB/2009.426), WHO, Switzerland, 2009

# Annex 5: Directory of partners for countries with a high-burden of TB

## Cambodia

**US Agency for International Development (USAID)**
#1, St. 96, Khan Daun Penh, Phnom Penh

**The Tuberculosis Control Assistance Program (TB CAP)**
National Center for TB and Leprosy services (CENAT)
St. 278–95, Beong Keng Kang II, Phnom Penh

**World Health Organization (WHO)**
177–179, St. Pasteur (St.51), Chak Tomouk, Phnom Penh

**Japan Anti-Tuberculosis Association (JATA)**
# 6, St. 288, Beong Keng Kang II, Phnom Penh

**Japan International Cooperation Agency (JICA)**
National Center for TB and Leprosy services (CENAT)
St. 278–95, Beong Keng Kang II, Phnom Penh

**University Research Co. (URC)**
Phnom Penh Center,
Second floor, Corner of Sihanouk & Sothearos Bld, Tonle Bassac, Phnom Penh

**Christian Action Research and Action (CARE)**
#52, W5 352, Phnom Penh

**Reproductive Health Association of Cambodia (RHAC)**
#6, St. 150, Sangat Veal Vong,
Phnom Penh

**Reproductive and Child Health Alliance (RACHA)**
#160, St. 71, Tonle Bassac,
Phnom Penh

**Cambodian Health Committee (CHC)**
#64, Street 592, Boeung Kok II, Tuol Kork, Phnom Penh
Dr. Thor Chanthe (chcsr@online.com.kh), TB Coordinator
855 (44) 945 820, 855 (11) 851 543, or 855 (23) 885 169

**Programme for Appropriate Technology in Health (PATH)**
#22, St. 184, Phnom Penh

**Family Health International (FHI)**
# 11, St. 302, Boeung Keng Kang, Phnom Penh
ngak@fhi.org.kh, caroline@fhi.org.kh
Tel: 855 – 023 211914/212565

**US-Centers for Disease Control and Prevention**
National Institute of Public Health, P.O Box 1300, Phnom Penh

**Catholic Relief Services (CRS) in partnership with AHEAD (Action for Health and Development)**
#14, St. 278, S/K Beung Keng Kang I,
Phnom Penh
bunsieth@online.com.kh
Tel: 012 -907 802

**Health And Development Alliance, HEAD**
House #00, Klang Prak Village,
Khum Pha Ear, Kampong Chhnang District,
Kampong Chhnang province
ch-sopha@camintel.com
Tel: +855 12 989 242 or +855 16 857 275

**Health Unlimited (HU)**
# 37, St. 396, Boeung Keng kang 3,
Chamcarmon, Phnom Penh
Ms. Khou Somatheavy
(khousomatheavy@everyday.com.kh),
Country Manager
Mr. Sam Ossophea
(humco@everyday.com.kh),
Program Coordinator
Tel/Fax 023 215192 / 214363

**Partners For Health and Development, PFHAD**
Phsa Veng village, Kratie Commune,
Kratie District, Kratie Province
p_pfhaded@hellogsm.com.kh
Tel: 012 366 075

**RHAC (Reproductive Health Association of Cambodia)**
# 14, St. 317, Sangkat Boeung Kak 1,
Khan Tuol Kork, Phnom Penh
chivorn@rhac.org.kh
Tel 023 885 135, Mobile : 012 982 294

**Save the Children Australia (SCA)**
Mr Hang Vuthy, SCA Kampong Cham Office,
012 830 162, hssp_om@sca-cambodia.org
Ms Carol Mortensen, #51, Street 352, Phnom Penh, 012 833 603, cpd@sca-cambodia.org

**Sihanouk Hospital Centre of HOPE (SHCH)**
1/ Street 134, Sangkat Vealvong, Khan 7 Makara, Phnom Penh
sopheakthai2003@yahoo.com, gerlinda_lucas@online.com.kh
Tel 011 842 034, 011 716 704,

**VOR ORT**
P.O.Box 89008, 16000 Ratanakiri Province
tb@vorortev.org
075 97 40 67, 012 78 59 33

**Cambodia Anti-Tuberculosis Association (CATA)**
P.O Box: 2589, CCC Box: 364
c/o CENAT, 278/95, S/K Beoung Keng Kang II,
Khan Chamka morn, Phnom Penh
cata_cambodia@yahoo.com ,
mom_ky011@yahoo.com
Tel: 023–218091, Fax/Tel: 855–23 218090,

## China

**Damien Foundation Belgium**
Rm 0601 Guangming Hotel, Liangmaqiao road, Beijing 100016
Jaucot Alex (alex.jaucot@damien-bel.org.cn)
Tel: (8610)84512250 ext 14
Fax: (8610)64637144
Focal areas: support DOTS implementation and MDR-TB in 5 provinces including Guizhou, Qinghai, NingXia, Tibet and Inner Mongolia

**China Medical Association, subgroup TB**
# 97 Machang, Tongzhou District, Beijing 101149
Fu Yu
Tel: (8610)69546690 ext 609
Fax: (8610)80882505
Focal areas: training, advocacy

**Bill and Melinda Gates Foundation**
Address: Room 1201, China resources Building, 8 Jiangguomenbei Avenue, Beijing 100005
Daniel P. Chin
(Daniel.chin@gatesfoundation.org)
Tel: (8610) 58111888
Fax: (8610) 58111999
Focal areas: MDR-TB (under negotiation)

**Clinton Foundation**
5–1–42 tayuan Diplomatic Office Bldg. #1
Xindong rd, beijing 100600
Herb Harwell (Herbhar@gmail.com)
Tel: (8610)85324950 ext 126
Fax: (8610)85324953
Focal areas: HIV and TB/HIV

**Bill and Melinda Gates Foundation**
Room 1201, China Resources Building,
8 Jiangguomenbei Avenue,
Beijing 100005
Daniel P. Chin
Daniel.chin@gatesfoundation.org
Tel: (8610) 58111888
Fax: (8610) 58111999

**World Bank**
16th floor, China World Tower 2. No.1
Jianguomenwai Avenue, Beijing 10004
Zhang Shuo (szhang2@worldbank.org)
Tel: (8610) 58617786
Fax: (8610) 58617800
Focal areas: basic DOTS in 16 provinces

**China Anti-TB Association**
# 27 Nanwei road, Xuanwu district,
Beijing 100050
DuanMu Hongjin (wanly@chinatb.org)
Tel: (8650) 83133137
Focal areas: training, advocacy, health education:

**All China Women's Association**
Focal areas: health education in villages (GF supported)

**DFID**
DFID China 30th floor South Tower, Kerry Centre, Chao Yang District, 1 Guang Hua Road,
Beijing 100020
Qiao Jianrong (jr-qiao@dfid.gov.uk)
Tel:+ 00 86 (0) 10 8529 6882
Fax:+ 00 86 (0) 10 8529 6002/3/4/5

## Lao People's Democratic Republic

**Damien Foundation Belgium (DFB)**
Dr Guido Groenen (guido.groenen@skynet.be)
DFB has provided technical support to NTP since DOTS start in 1995. DFB TB experts visit the country 2–3 times a year with focus on programme supervision and more recently on TB-HIV collaborative activities.

## Mongolia

**World Vision – international NGO**
1st khoroo, Sansar mega center "B" part, 5th floor, Ulaanbaatar, Mongolia
- Dr Amgalan Badamjav, TB project coordinator, amgalan_badamjav@wvi.org
- 976–70155323/976–70155322
- focal area: Prison and Enerel hospital, selected districts and provinces

**Mongolian Anti-tuberculosis Association**
Room 308, Building of "San" University, Bayangol district, Ulaanbaatar, Mongolia
- Dr Solongo Bekhbat, Executive Director (mvpho@magicnet.mn)
- 976–11–366617
- focal area: ACSM, food provision for TB patients, treatment follow up

## Papua New Guinea

**World Vision (Port Moresby)**
Mr Marlon Villanueva (marlon_villanueva@wvi.org)
focal area - ACSM component of the Stop TB Strategy

**HOPE worldwide (Port Moresby)**
Ms Jessica Lesley (jlesley@online.net.pg)
focal area - technical component of DOTS Strategy

**City Pharmacy (Port Moresby)**
Mr Sourav Mukherjee (sourav@cpl.com.pg)
focal area - procurement and supply management component

**JTA International (Port Moresby)**
Ms Ingrid Glastonbury
(ingrid.glastonbury@jtai.com.au)
focal area - monitoring and evaluation component

**WHO (Port Moresby)**
focal area - technical component of Stop TB Strategy

**PNG Institute of Medical Research (Goroka)**
Ms Geraldine.Maibani
(Geraldine.Maibani@pngimr.org.pg)
focal area - operational research

## Philippines

**Philippine Coalition Against Tuberculosis (PhilCAT)**
Quezon Institute
E. Rodriquez Avenue, Quezon City, Metro Manila
Ms Amelia Sarmiento, Executive Director
(agsarmiento@philcat.org)
Focal Area: Public-Private Mix for TB Care and Control

**RIT/JATA Philippines**
Tayuman Street and Rizal Ave corner,
2nd Floor, Santa Cruz, City of Manila,
Metro Manila
Dr Roderick Poblete
Focal Area: Urban Poor TB control

**World Vision Development Fund**
Quezon Avenue, Quezon City, Metro Manila
Ms. Ma. Imelda Ochavillo
(imelda_ochavillo@wvi.org)
Focal Area: ACSM

**Philippine Business for Social Progress (PBSP)**
Supported by USAID
Intramuros, City of Manila, Metro Manila
Focal Area: PPMD, TB in Children, TB Finance
e-mail: JAGutierrez@pbsp.org.ph

## Viet Nam

**Embassy of Netherlands**
Daeha Office Tower,
6th Floor, 360 Kim Ma Street, Hanoi
Tel 84.4.38315650, Fax 84.4.38315655

**CDC**
Rose Garden, 6 Ngoc Khanh Street, Hanoi
Dr Bruce Baird Struminger
(strumingerbb@vn.cdc.gov),
Country Director
Tel 84.4.38314604, Fax 84.4.38314580

**US Embassy**
7 Lang Ha Street, Hanoi
Dr Michael Iademarco (iademarcoMF@state.gov),
Health Attaché
Tel 84.4.38314580, Fax 84.4.38505028

**USAID**
15/F Tung Shing Square,
#2 Ngo Quyen Street, Hanoi
Mrs. Ellen Lynch
Tel 84.4.39351265

# Annex 6: Explanatory notes for tables

Regional summary and country and territory data are presented in the following 10 tables. All rates are per 100 000 population.

**Table 47:**
**Estimated burden of TB, 2000 and 2008**
Estimates of incidence, prevalence and mortality for 2000 (baseline year for impact goal endorsed by the Regional Committee) and 2008 (the latest year covered by this report). See Annexes 4 for details of calculations. All estimates include TB in people living with human immunodeficiency virus (HIV).

**Table 48:**
**Whole country and area case notifications and case detection rates, 2008**
Case notifications by history (new or retreatment), by site (pulmonary or extrapulmonary) and by smear status (smear-positive, smear-negative, or unknown). Proportions of case types and estimated case detection rate for whole country and territory .

- *Population, source: World Population Prospects: The 2008 Revision*. New York: United Nations Population Division, 2009.
- *WHO total:* new and relapse cases.
- *New pulmonary ss+:* new pulmonary cases in which diagnosis has been confirmed by smear examination.
- *New pulmonary ss-/unk.:* new pulmonary cases in which diagnosis has not been confirmed by smear examination or the result is unknown.
- *New extrapulmonary:* new extrapulmonary cases.
- *Other new:* new cases for which the site of disease is not recorded.
- *Other re-treat.:* retreatment cases for which the outcome of previous treatment is unknown.
- *Other:* cases for which neither treatment history nor site of disease is recorded.
- *New pulm. lab. confirm.:* new pulmonary cases in which diagnosis has been confirmed by smear and/or culture examination.
- *Case detection rate, all new:* notified (new and relapse) cases divided by estimated incident cases (expressed as a percentage).
- *ss+ (% of pulm.):* the percentage of all new pulmonary cases that are smear-positive.
- *ss+ (% of new+relapse):* the percentage of new and relapse cases that are smear-positive.
- *Extrapulm. (% of new+relapse):* the percentage of all new and relapse cases that are extrapulmonary.
- *Re-treat. (% of new+re-treat.):* notified retreatment cases as a percentage of all notified cases.

**Table 49:**
**Laboratory services, management of MDR-TB, and collaborative TB-HIV activities**
**Laboratory services**

- *Number of laboratories:* the number of laboratories working with the national TB control programme (NTP) that perform smear microscopy, culture or anti-TB drug susceptibility testing (DST), and the number of laboratories performing smear microscopy that are included in external quality assessment (EQA).

**MDR-TB, 2008**

- *Lab-confirmed MDR among new & retreatment cases:* number of laboratory-confirmed cases of multidrug-resistant (MDR)-TB identified among TB patients (new and retreatment) diagnosed in 2008.
- *DST in new cases:* number of new TB cases in 2008 for which DST was performed at start of treatment.
- *MDR in new cases:* number of new cases identified as MDR-TB based on DST at start of treatment.
- *Retreatment with DST:* number of retreatment cases registered in 2008 for which DST was performed at start of treatment.

- *Re-treat. MDR:* number of retreatment cases identified as MDR-TB based on DST at start of treatment.

**Collaborative TB-HIV activities, 2007 and 2008**

- *TB patients tested for HIV:* the number of TB patients tested for HIV.
- *Of those tested, HIV positive:* the number of TB patients found to be HIV-positive.
- *Of those HIV positive, started co-trimoxazole:* the number of HIV-positive TB patients given CPT.
- *Of those HIV positive, started antiretroviral therapy (ART):* the number of HIV-positive TB patients given ART during their TB treatment.

**Table 50:**
**Treatment outcomes, 2007 cohort**
Treatment outcomes of new smear-positive cases treated under DOTS and retreatment cases under DOTS.

**Table 51:**
**DOTS treatment success and case detection rates, 1994–2008**
Treatment success rates (the proportion of registered cases cured or completed treatment) for new smear-positive cases treated under DOTS from 1994 to 2007 and all forms case detection rates from 1995 to 2008.

**Table 52:**
**New smear-positive case notification by age and sex, absolute numbers, 2008**
Breakdown by age and sex of new smear-positive cases notified by country and territory. Some countries and areas cannot provide the breakdown for all notified smear-positive cases.

**Table 53:**
**New smear-positive case notification rates by age and sex, 2008**
Notification rates of new smear-positive cases by age and sex. Rates are missing where breakdown of smear-positive notified cases is not provided, or if age- and sex-specific population data are not available. In the regional summary row, rates exclude those countries for which breakdown of notified cases or population by age and sex is missing.

**Table 54:**
**Number of TB cases notified, 1980–2008**

**Table 55:**
**Case notification rates, 1980–2008**

**Table 56:**
**New smear-positive cases notified, numbers and rates, 1993–2008**

# Annex 7: Tables

**Table 47.** Estimated burden of TB, 2000 and 2008

| | Incidence, 2000 | | | | Prevalence, 2000 | | TB mortality, 2000 | | Incidence, 2008 | | | |
|---|---|---|---|---|---|---|---|---|---|---|---|---|
| | All forms* | | Smear-positive* | | All forms* | | All forms* | | All forms* | | All forms HIV+ | |
| | number | rate | number | rate | number | rate | number | rate | number | rate | number | rate |
| American Samoa | 3 | 6 | 2 | 3 | 1 | 2 | | | 2 | 3 | 2 | 3 |
| Australia | 1200 | 6 | 290 | 2 | 750 | 4 | 35 | | 1400 | 7 | 33 | |
| Brunei Darussalam | 350 | 110 | 97 | 29 | 330 | 98 | 16 | 5 | 260 | 65 | | |
| Cambodia | 68 000 | 530 | 33 000 | 260 | 130 000 | 1000 | 14 000 | 110 | 71 000 | 490 | 11 000 | 73 |
| China | 1 300 000 | 110 | 660 000 | 52 | 2 700 000 | 210 | 320 000 | 25 | 1 300 000 | 97 | 22 000 | 2 |
| Cook Islands | 1 | 7 | 1 | 3 | 1 | 3 | | | 4 | 20 | | |
| Fiji | 240 | 30 | 120 | 15 | 240 | 30 | 32 | 4 | 170 | 20 | 6 | 1 |
| French Polynesia | 71 | 30 | 33 | 14 | 18 | 8 | 4 | 2 | 58 | 22 | | |
| Guam | 62 | 40 | 49 | 32 | 30 | 19 | 4 | 3 | 100 | 58 | 3 | 2 |
| Hong Kong (China) | 6900 | 100 | 2200 | 33 | 3800 | 58 | 440 | 7 | 6400 | 91 | 32 | |
| Japan | 45 000 | 36 | 14 000 | 11 | 29 000 | 23 | 2800 | 2 | 28 000 | 22 | 140 | |
| Kiribati | 350 | 420 | 170 | 210 | 420 | 490 | 54 | 64 | 350 | 360 | | |
| Lao People's Democratic Republic | 8700 | 160 | 4300 | 80 | 19 000 | 360 | 2300 | 42 | 9300 | 150 | 190 | 3 |
| Macao (China) | 520 | 120 | 180 | 42 | 300 | 68 | 32 | 7 | 410 | 78 | 1 | |
| Malaysia | 25 000 | 110 | 13 000 | 54 | 33 000 | 140 | 4000 | 17 | 28 000 | 100 | 3 400 | 12 |
| Marshall Islands | 130 | 250 | 64 | 120 | 270 | 510 | 31 | 60 | 130 | 210 | | |
| Federated States of Micronesia | 140 | 130 | 68 | 63 | 140 | 130 | 19 | 17 | 100 | 93 | | |
| Mongolia | 4900 | 210 | 2400 | 100 | 5500 | 230 | 720 | 30 | 5400 | 210 | 8 | |
| Nauru | 4 | 44 | 2 | 22 | 5 | 50 | 1 | 7 | 1 | 12 | | |
| New Caledonia | 110 | 50 | 23 | 11 | 110 | 51 | 8 | 4 | 51 | 21 | | |
| New Zealand | 400 | 10 | 85 | 2 | 120 | 3 | 12 | | 340 | 8 | 3 | |
| Niue | | | | | | 4 | | | | | | |
| Commonwealth of the Northern Mariana Islands | 86 | 120 | 31 | 45 | 75 | 110 | 6 | 8 | 32 | 38 | | |
| Palau | 10 | 52 | 5 | 26 | 5 | 23 | 1 | 4 | 13 | 63 | | |
| Papua New Guinea | 13 000 | 250 | 6600 | 120 | 7000 | 130 | 1200 | 21 | 16 000 | 250 | 620 | 9 |
| Philippines | 260 000 | 330 | 130 000 | 160 | 600 000 | 780 | 51 000 | 66 | 260 000 | 280 | 660 | 1 |
| Republic of Korea | 25 000 | 54 | 9400 | 20 | 7600 | 16 | 4100 | 9 | 42 000 | 88 | 220 | |
| Samoa | 41 | 23 | 20 | 12 | 35 | 20 | 5 | 3 | 33 | 18 | | |
| Singapore | 2000 | 49 | 290 | 7 | 1300 | 32 | 130 | 3 | 1800 | 39 | 45 | 1 |
| Solomon Islands | 770 | 180 | 380 | 91 | 1500 | 360 | 180 | 43 | 620 | 120 | | |
| Tokelau | | | | | | | | | | | | |
| Tonga | 27 | 28 | 13 | 14 | 28 | 29 | 4 | 4 | 24 | 24 | | |
| Tuvalu | 20 | 210 | 10 | 100 | 18 | 190 | 3 | 26 | 16 | 160 | | |
| Vanuatu | 190 | 98 | 92 | 49 | 150 | 79 | 21 | 11 | 170 | 74 | | |
| Viet Nam | 160 000 | 200 | 79 000 | 100 | 230 000 | 290 | 28 000 | 36 | 170 000 | 200 | 6 600 | 7 |
| Wallis and Futuna | 8 | 52 | 4 | 25 | 20 | 140 | 2 | 16 | 1 | 6 | | |
| **Western Pacific Region** | **1 923 234** | **114** | **955 928** | **57** | **3 770 765** | **224** | **429 158** | **26** | **1 942 185** | **109** | **44 964** | **2** |

* Incidence, prevalence and mortality estimates include patients with HIV. Estimates labelled "HIV+" are estimates of TB in HIV-positive adults (age 15–49). Estimates for all years are re-calculated as new information becomes available and techniques are refined, so they may differ from those published previously. See Explanatory notes on page 62 for further details. Data can be downloaded from http://stoptb.wpro.who.int.

| Incidence, 2008 | | Prevalence, 2008 | | TB mortality, 2008 | | HIV prevalence in adult incident TB cases (%) | |
|---|---|---|---|---|---|---|---|
| Smear-positive* | | All forms* | | All forms* | | | |
| number | rate | number | rate | number | rate | | |
| 1 | 2 | 1 | 1 | | 0 | 100 | American Samoa |
| 340 | 2 | 940 | 5 | 89 | 0 | 2.3 | Australia |
| 150 | 39 | 170 | 43 | 17 | 4 | 0 | Brunei Darussalam |
| 35 000 | 240 | 99 000 | 680 | 11 000 | 79 | 15 | Cambodia |
| 640 000 | 48 | 1 200 000 | 88 | 160 000 | 12 | 1.7 | China |
| 2 | 10 | 6 | 32 | 1 | 4 | | Cook Islands |
| 82 | 10 | 210 | 25 | 27 | 3 | 3.3 | Fiji |
| 23 | 9 | 15 | 6 | 4 | 1 | | French Polynesia |
| 36 | 20 | 110 | 61 | 7 | 4 | 3.3 | Guam |
| 1700 | 24 | 4000 | 58 | 410 | 6 | 0.51 | Hong Kong (China) |
| 10 000 | 8 | 16 000 | 12 | 1800 | 1 | 0.49 | Japan |
| 170 | 180 | 110 | 110 | 24 | 25 | 0 | Kiribati |
| 4600 | 74 | 16 000 | 260 | 2000 | 32 | 2 | Lao People's Democratic Republic |
| 160 | 30 | 260 | 49 | 26 | 5 | 0.25 | Macao (China) |
| 14 000 | 51 | 34 000 | 120 | 4000 | 15 | 12 | Malaysia |
| 63 | 100 | 36 | 59 | 8 | 14 | 0 | Marshall Islands |
| 51 | 46 | 38 | 34 | 7 | 7 | 0 | Federated States of Micronesia |
| 2700 | 100 | 3600 | 140 | 540 | 21 | 0.15 | Mongolia |
| 1 | 6 | 1 | 10 | | 1 | | Nauru |
| 10 | 4 | 25 | 10 | 3 | 1 | | New Caledonia |
| 120 | 3 | 220 | 5 | 22 | 1 | 1 | New Zealand |
| | | | | | 0 | | Niue |
| 15 | 18 | 9 | 11 | 2 | 2 | 0 | Commonwealth of the Northern Mariana Islands |
| 6 | 31 | 23 | 110 | 3 | 14 | | Palau |
| 8100 | 120 | 8600 | 130 | 1400 | 21 | 3.8 | Papua New Guinea |
| 130 000 | 140 | 490 000 | 550 | 47 000 | 52 | 0.26 | Philippines |
| 13 000 | 26 | 24 000 | 50 | 2700 | 6 | 0.53 | Republic of Korea |
| 16 | 9 | 64 | 36 | 8 | 4 | | Samoa |
| 600 | 13 | 1300 | 27 | 110 | 3 | 2.5 | Singapore |
| 310 | 60 | 750 | 150 | 97 | 19 | | Solomon Islands |
| | | | | | 0 | | Tokelau |
| 12 | 12 | 23 | 22 | 3 | 3 | 0 | Tonga |
| 8 | 79 | 4 | 44 | 1 | 11 | 0 | Tuvalu |
| 86 | 37 | 210 | 88 | 27 | 11 | | Vanuatu |
| 86 000 | 99 | 240 000 | 280 | 30 000 | 34 | 3.8 | Viet Nam |
| | 3 | | 2 | | 0 | | Wallis and Futuna |
| **947 362** | **53** | **2 139 726** | **120** | **261 336** | **15** | **2.3** | **Western Pacific Region** |

**Table 48.** Whole country and area case notifications and case detection rates, 2008

| | Population thousands | New and relapse (WHO total) | | New pulmonary ss+ | | New pulmonary ss-/unk. | New extra-pulmonary | Other new | Retreatment cases | |
|---|---|---|---|---|---|---|---|---|---|---|
| | | number | rate | number | rate | number | number | number | Relapse number | After failure number |
| American Samoa | 67 | 3 | 5 | | | 3 | | | | |
| Australia | 21 074 | 1213 | 6 | 299 | 1 | 409 | 473 | 1 | 31 | |
| Brunei Darussalam | 392 | 223 | 57 | 132 | 34 | 28 | 43 | 8 | 12 | |
| Cambodia | 14 562 | 38 927 | 267 | 19 860 | 136 | 7847 | 10 678 | | 542 | 50 |
| China | 1 337 411 | 975 821 | 73 | 462 596 | 35 | 431 115 | 35 546 | 2863 | 43 701 | 2162 |
| Cook Islands | 20 | 2 | 10 | 2 | 10 | | | | | |
| Fiji | 844 | 106 | 13 | 78 | 9 | 5 | 19 | | 4 | |
| French Polynesia | 266 | 50 | 19 | 20 | 8 | 18 | 10 | | 2 | |
| Guam | 176 | 89 | 51 | 31 | 18 | 50 | 8 | | | |
| Hong Kong (China) | 6982 | 5544 | 79 | 1459 | 21 | 2981 | 728 | | 376 | 2 |
| Japan | 127 293 | 24 181 | 19 | 8995 | 7 | 8856 | 5073 | | 1257 | |
| Kiribati | 110 | 335 | 304 | 147 | 133 | 71 | 107 | | 10 | 1 |
| Lao People's Democratic Republic | 6205 | 4048 | 65 | 3079 | 53 | 519 | 298 | | 152 | 11 |
| Macao (China) | 526 | 359 | 68 | 139 | 29 | 150 | 49 | | 21 | |
| Malaysia | 27 014 | 17 144 | 63 | 10 441 | 39 | 3814 | 2197 | | 692 | 23 |
| Marshall Islands | 61 | 125 | 206 | 28 | 46 | 62 | 30 | | 5 | |
| Federated States of Micronesia | 97 | 164 | 169 | 38 | 39 | 89 | 30 | 4 | 3 | |
| Mongolia | 2641 | 4490 | 170 | 1838 | 70 | 640 | 1745 | | 267 | 81 |
| Nauru | 10 | 5 | 50 | 2 | 20 | 2 | | | 1 | |
| New Caledonia | 246 | 44 | 18 | 9 | 4 | 22 | 10 | | 3 | |
| New Zealand | 4230 | 292 | 7 | 101 | 2 | 91 | 92 | 2 | 6 | |
| Niue | 1 | 0 | 0 | 0 | 0 | 0 | | | | |
| Commonwealth of the Northern Mariana Islands | 85 | 28 | 33 | 13 | 15 | 12 | 3 | | | |
| Palau | 21 | | | | | | | | | |
| Papua New Guinea | 6577 | 13 984 | 213 | 2323 | 35 | 5340 | 4522 | | 1799 | |
| Philippines | 90 348 | 139 603 | 155 | 85 025 | 94 | 49 916 | 2085 | | 2577 | 522 |
| Republic of Korea | 48 152 | 36 847 | 77 | 11 048 | 23 | 17 292 | 5813 | | 2694 | 148 |
| Samoa | 179 | 12 | 7 | 6 | 3 | 5 | 1 | | | |
| Singapore | 4615 | 1549 | 34 | 526 | 11 | 672 | 240 | | 111 | 2 |
| Solomon Islands | 511 | 387 | 76 | 140 | 27 | 136 | 97 | | 14 | |
| Tokelau | 1 | 0 | 0 | 0 | | 0 | | | | |
| Tonga | 104 | 13 | 13 | 11 | 11 | | 2 | | | |
| Tuvalu | 10 | 17 | 170 | 9 | 90 | 5 | 3 | | | 1 |
| Vanuatu | 234 | 103 | 44 | 45 | 19 | 19 | 39 | | | |
| Viet Nam | 87 096 | 97 772 | 112 | 53 484 | 61 | 19 056 | 18 610 | | 6622 | 583 |
| Wallis and Futuna | 15 | | | | | | | | | |
| **Western Pacific Region** | **1 788 175** | **1 363 480** | **76** | **661 924** | **37** | **549 225** | **88 551** | **2878** | **60 902** | **3586** |

ss+ = sputum smear-positive; ss- = sputum smear-negative; unk. = sputum smear result unknown; re-treat. = retreatment; pulm. lab. confirm. = pulmonary case confirmed by positive smear or culture. See Explanatory notes on page 62 for further details. Data can be downloaded from http://stoptb.wpro.who.int.

| Retreatment cases | | | | Incidence and case detection rates | | | Proportions | | | | |
|---|---|---|---|---|---|---|---|---|---|---|---|
| | | | | Estimated incidence | | Case detection rate | | | | | |
| After default number | Other re-treat. number | Other number | New pulm. lab. con-firm. | all forms number | ss+ number | all new % | ss+ (% of pulm.) | ss+ (% of new+ relapse) | Extrapulm. (% of new+ relapse) | Re-treat. (% of new+ re-treat.) | |
| | | | | 2 | 1 | 140 | 0 | 0 | 0 | 0 | American Samoa |
| 4 | 8 | 2 | 656 | 1 400 | 340 | 87 | 42 | 27 | 39 | 4 | Australia |
| | | 2 | 159 | 260 | 150 | 87 | 83 | 67 | 20 | 5 | Brunei Darussalam |
| 20 | 823 | | 27 707 | 71 000 | 35 000 | 55 | 72 | 52 | 27 | 4 | Cambodia |
| 2174 | 54 042 | | 462 596 | 1 300 000 | 640 000 | 75 | 52 | 52 | 4 | 10 | China |
| | | | 2 | 4 | 2 | 50 | 100 | 100 | 0 | 0 | Cook Islands |
| | | | 78 | 170 | 82 | 64 | 94 | 77 | 18 | 4 | Fiji |
| | | | 37 | 58 | 23 | 87 | 53 | 44 | 20 | 4 | French Polynesia |
| | 1 | | 35 | 100 | 36 | 87 | 38 | 35 | 9 | 1 | Guam |
| 32 | 151 | | 3210 | 6 400 | 1 700 | 87 | 33 | 33 | 13 | 10 | Hong Kong (China) |
| | 579 | | 14 625 | 28 000 | 10 000 | 87 | 50 | 42 | 21 | 7 | Japan |
| | 6 | | 147 | 350 | 170 | 97 | 67 | 47 | 32 | 5 | Kiribati |
| 17 | | 76 | 3896 | 9 300 | 4 600 | 44 | 86 | 80 | 7 | 4 | Lao People's Democratic Republic |
| 2 | 15 | 35 | 247 | 410 | 160 | 87 | 48 | 45 | 14 | 10 | Macao (China) |
| 339 | | | 14 767 | 28 000 | 14 000 | 62 | 73 | 65 | 13 | 6 | Malaysia |
| 1 | 1 | | 28 | 130 | 63 | 98 | 31 | 26 | 24 | 6 | Marshall Islands |
| 2 | | | 38 | 100 | 51 | 160 | 30 | 26 | 19 | 3 | Federated States of Micronesia |
| 37 | 159 | | 1838 | 5 400 | 2 700 | 83 | 74 | 47 | 39 | 11 | Mongolia |
| 1 | 1 | | 2 | 1 | 1 | 420 | 50 | 60 | 0 | 43 | Nauru |
| | 1 | 6 | 25 | 51 | 10 | 87 | 29 | 27 | 23 | 9 | New Caledonia |
| | 5 | | 173 | 340 | 120 | 87 | 53 | 37 | 32 | 4 | New Zealand |
| | | | | | | | | | | | Niue |
| | 2 | | 13 | 32 | 15 | 87 | 52 | 46 | 11 | 7 | Commonwealth of the Northern Mariana Islands |
| | | | | 13 | 6 | 0 | | | | | Palau |
| | | | 4979 | 16 000 | 8 100 | 85 | 30 | 29 | 32 | 13 | Papua New Guinea |
| 720 | 5047 | | 88 682 | 260 000 | 130 000 | 54 | 63 | 63 | 1 | 6 | Philippines |
| 378 | 3090 | 3707 | 16 421 | 42 000 | 13 000 | 87 | 39 | 37 | 16 | 16 | Republic of Korea |
| | | | 12 | 33 | 16 | 37 | 55 | 50 | 8 | 0 | Samoa |
| 2 | 36 | 13 | 951 | 1 800 | 600 | 87 | 44 | 41 | 15 | 10 | Singapore |
| | | | 140 | 620 | 310 | 63 | 51 | 40 | 25 | 4 | Solomon Islands |
| | | | | | | | | | | | Tokelau |
| | | | 11 | 24 | 12 | 53 | 100 | 85 | 15 | 0 | Tonga |
| 1 | | | 9 | 16 | 8 | 110 | 64 | 53 | 18 | 11 | Tuvalu |
| 1 | | | 45 | 170 | 86 | 59 | 70 | 44 | 38 | 1 | Vanuatu |
| 329 | | | 61 588 | 170 000 | 86 000 | 56 | 74 | 61 | 19 | 8 | Viet Nam |
| | | | | 1 | | 0 | | | | | Wallis and Futuna |
| **4060** | **63 967** | **3841** | **703 117** | **1 942 185** | **947 362** | **70** | **55** | **53** | **7** | **9** | **Western Pacific Region** |

**Table 49.** Laboratory services, management of MDR-TB and collaborative TB-HIV activities

| | Laboratory services | | | | | Multidrug-resistant TB, 2008 | | | | |
|---|---|---|---|---|---|---|---|---|---|---|
| | Number of laboratories | | | Laboratories included in EQA | Laboratories with performance un-acceptable | Lab-confirmed MDR among new & re-treat. cases number | DST in new cases number | MDR in new cases number | Re-treat. with DST number | Re-treat. MDR number |
| | smear | culture | DST | | | | | | | |
| American Samoa | | | | | | | | | | |
| Australia | | | | | | 19 | 896 | 15 | 33 | 4 |
| Brunei Darussalam | 1 | 1 | 1 | 1 | | | | | | |
| Cambodia | 202 | 3 | 1 | 202 | | 31 | 11 | 3 | 91 | 28 |
| China | 3294 | 628 | 109 | 3294 | 14 | | | | | |
| Cook Islands | | | | | | | | | | |
| Fiji | 4 | 1 | | | | | | | | |
| French Polynesia | 2 | 2 | 2 | 2 | | | 46 | | 2 | |
| Guam | 2 | 1 | 1 | | | | 37 | | | |
| Hong Kong (China) | 26 | 20 | 3 | 21 | | 28 | 3121 | 14 | 390 | 14 |
| Japan | | | | | | | | | | |
| Kiribati | | | | | | | | | | |
| Lao People's Democratic Republic | 155 | | | 154 | 9 | | | | | |
| Macao (China) | 8 | 1 | | 1 | 1 | 7 | 243 | 5 | 25 | 2 |
| Malaysia | 656 | 14 | 3 | 277 | 1 | 56 | | | | |
| Marshall Islands | | | | | | | | | | |
| Federated States of Micronesia | 8 | | | 4 | | 4 | 40 | 4 | 3 | |
| Mongolia | 36 | 1 | 1 | 36 | | 115 | 75 | 1 | 334 | 114 |
| Nauru | | | | | | | | | | |
| New Caledonia | | | | | | | 41 | | 4 | |
| New Zealand | | | | | | | 231 | | 11 | |
| Niue | | | | | | | | | | |
| Commonwealth of the Northern Mariana Islands | 1 | 1 | 1 | 1 | | | | | | |
| Palau | | | | | | | | | | |
| Papua New Guinea | 111 | 1 | 1 | 40 | 17 | 5 | | | | |
| Philippines | 2374 | 3 | 3 | 1925 | | 929 | 74 | 14 | 1305 | 729 |
| Republic of Korea | 260 | 12 | 7 | 1 | | | | | | |
| Samoa | 2 | | | 1 | 1 | | | | | |
| Singapore | | | | | | 4 | 919 | 1 | 103 | 3 |
| Solomon Islands | 9 | | | 9 | | | | | | |
| Tokelau | | | | | | | | | | |
| Tonga | 1 | 1 | | 1 | 1 | | | | | |
| Tuvalu | 1 | | | 1 | | | | | | |
| Vanuatu | 5 | | | 5 | 2 | | | | | |
| Viet Nam | 809 | 30 | 2 | 809 | | | | | | |
| Wallis and Futuna | | | | | | | | | | |
| **Western Pacific Region** | | | | | | **1198** | **5734** | **57** | **2301** | **894** |

ART = antiretroviral treatment; BMU = basic management unit; DST = drug susceptibility testing; EQA = external quality assessment; MDR = multidrug-resistant; re-treat. = retreatment.
Laboratory data was not collected from high-income countries and most Pacific island countries.

| Collaborative TB/HIV activities | | | | | | | | |
|---|---|---|---|---|---|---|---|---|
| 2006 | | | | 2007 | | | | |
| TB patients tested for HIV | Of those tested, HIV positive | Of those HIV positive, started cotrimoxazole | Of those HIV positive, started ART | TB patients tested for HIV | Of those tested, HIV positive | Of those HIV positive, started cotrimoxazole | Of those HIV positive, started ART | |
| 3 | | | | 3 | | | | American Samoa |
| 575 | 20 | 3 | 10 | 725 | 17 | 2 | 10 | Australia |
| 209 | | | | 223 | | | | Brunei Darussalam |
| 17 105 | 5782 | 1101 | 610 | 21 523 | 3309 | 1279 | 733 | Cambodia |
| 67 265 | 1523 | 679 | 519 | 81 682 | 2848 | 1549 | 564 | China |
| | | | | | | | | Cook Islands |
| 57 | | | | 51 | | | | Fiji |
| 19 | | | | 16 | | | | French Polynesia |
| 58 | | | | 60 | 2 | | 1 | Guam |
| 4075 | 41 | 26 | 27 | 4121 | 48 | 16 | 19 | Hong Kong (China) |
| 16 100 | 57 | | | 13 777 | 67 | | | Japan |
| | | | | | | | | Kiribati |
| 469 | 196 | 182 | 61 | 557 | 221 | 217 | 130 | Lao People's Democratic Republic |
| 360 | 4 | | 1 | 376 | 1 | | | Macao (China) |
| 10 082 | 1629 | | 72 | 14 726 | 1819 | | 791 | Malaysia |
| 98 | | | | 82 | | | | Marshall Islands |
| 44 | | | | 64 | | | | Federated States of Micronesia |
| 1450 | 3 | 1 | 1 | 1296 | 1 | 1 | 1 | Mongolia |
| | | | | | | | | Nauru |
| | | | | | | | | New Caledonia |
| 104 | 4 | | | 138 | 8 | | | New Zealand |
| | | | | | | | | Niue |
| 41 | | | | 35 | | | | Commonwealth of the Northern Mariana Islands |
| | | | | | | | | Palau |
| 117 | | 27 | 320 | 582 | | 1444 | 555 | Papua New Guinea |
| 46 | | | | 1069 | | | | Philippines |
| | | | | | | | | Republic of Korea |
| | | | | | | | | Samoa |
| | | | | | | | | Singapore |
| 3 | | | | | | | | Solomon Islands |
| | | | | | | | | Tokelau |
| 23 | | | | 13 | | | | Tonga |
| | | | | 17 | | | | Tuvalu |
| | | | | | | | | Vanuatu |
| 5495 | 1431 | | | 11 332 | 2210 | 1724 | 701 | Viet Nam |
| | | | | | | | | Wallis and Futuna |
| **123 798** | **10 690** | **2019** | **1621** | **152 468** | **10 551** | **6232** | **3505** | **Western Pacific Region** |

**Table 50.** Treatment outcomes, 2007 cohort

| | New smear-positive cases, DOTS | | | | | | | | | | |
|---|---|---|---|---|---|---|---|---|---|---|---|
| | Number of cases | | % of notif regist'd | % of cohort | | | | | | | % Success |
| | Notified | Regist'd | | Cured | Completed | Died | Failed | Default | Trans-ferred | Not eval. | |
| American Samoa | | | | | | | | | | | |
| Australia | 498 | 498 | 100 | 7 | 77 | 6 | 0 | 2 | 5 | 2 | 85 |
| Brunei Darussalam | 136 | 136 | 100 | 63 | 13 | 4 | 0 | 2 | 18 | 0 | 76 |
| Cambodia | 19 429 | 19 429 | 100 | 91 | 3 | 3 | 0 | 1 | 1 | 1 | 94 |
| China | 465 877 | 465 877 | 100 | 93 | 2 | 1 | 1 | 1 | 3 | 0 | 94 |
| Cook Islands | 2 | 2 | 100 | 0 | 100 | 0 | 0 | 0 | 0 | 0 | 100 |
| Fiji | 78 | 78 | 100 | 81 | 0 | 5 | 0 | 10 | 4 | 0 | 81 |
| French Polynesia | 26 | 26 | 100 | 85 | 0 | 12 | 0 | 4 | 0 | 0 | 85 |
| Guam | 36 | 36 | 100 | 89 | 0 | 6 | 0 | 0 | 6 | 0 | 89 |
| Hong Kong (China) | 1481 | 1481 | 100 | 59 | 7 | 11 | 14 | 6 | 3 | 0 | 66 |
| Japan | 9421 | 9421 | 100 | 17 | 29 | 18 | 1 | 5 | 3 | 27 | 46 |
| Kiribati | 100 | 100 | 100 | 79 | 14 | 7 | 0 | 0 | 0 | 0 | 93 |
| Lao People's Democratic Republic | 3080 | 3080 | 100 | 91 | 2 | 6 | 0 | 1 | 0 | 0 | 92 |
| Macao (China) | 251 | 251 | 100 | 49 | 42 | 6 | 0 | 1 | 2 | 0 | 91 |
| Malaysia | 10 236 | 10 236 | 100 | 67 | 5 | 8 | 0 | 5 | 6 | 9 | 72 |
| Marshall Islands | 27 | 27 | 100 | 93 | 4 | 0 | 0 | 4 | 0 | 0 | 96 |
| Federated States of Micronesia | 52 | 52 | 100 | 25 | 40 | 8 | 2 | 4 | 4 | 17 | 65 |
| Mongolia | 1855 | 1855 | 100 | 85 | 4 | 2 | 6 | 2 | 0 | 0 | 89 |
| Nauru | 2 | 2 | 100 | 0 | 100 | 0 | 0 | 0 | 0 | 0 | 100 |
| New Caledonia | 13 | 13 | 100 | 69 | 8 | 23 | 0 | 0 | 0 | 0 | 77 |
| New Zealand | 84 | 84 | 100 | 0 | 86 | 7 | 0 | 1 | 5 | 1 | 86 |
| Niue | | | | | | | | | | | |
| Commonwealth of the Northern Mariana Islands | 13 | 13 | 100 | 0 | 92 | 0 | 0 | 0 | 8 | 0 | 92 |
| Palau | | | | | | | | | | | |
| Papua New Guinea | 2087 | 2087 | 100 | 33 | 6 | 1 | 2 | 6 | 2 | 49 | 39 |
| Philippines | 86 566 | 86 566 | 100 | 79 | 10 | 2 | 1 | 4 | 3 | 1 | 89 |
| Republic of Korea | 3987 | 3987 | 100 | 81 | 1 | 1 | 1 | 4 | 12 | 0 | 82 |
| Samoa | 13 | 13 | 100 | 85 | 8 | 0 | 8 | 0 | 0 | 0 | 92 |
| Singapore | 859 | 859 | 100 | 62 | 19 | 16 | 0 | 1 | 0 | 0 | 81 |
| Solomon Islands | 142 | 142 | 100 | 75 | 17 | 6 | 0 | 1 | 1 | 0 | 92 |
| Tokelau | | | | | | | | | | | |
| Tonga | 14 | 14 | 100 | 93 | 0 | 7 | 0 | 0 | 0 | 0 | 93 |
| Tuvalu | 16 | 16 | 100 | 56 | 19 | 13 | 0 | 6 | 6 | 0 | 75 |
| Vanuatu | 42 | 42 | 100 | 81 | 12 | 2 | 0 | 0 | 5 | 0 | 93 |
| Viet Nam | 54 457 | 54 457 | 100 | 89 | 2 | 3 | 1 | 2 | 2 | 0 | 92 |
| Wallis and Futuna | | | | | | | | | | | |
| **Western Pacific Region** | **660 880** | **660 880** | **100** | **89** | **3** | **2** | **1** | **1** | **3** | **1** | **92** |

Not eval. = not evaluated (percentage of registered cases for which outcomes were not recorded); success = sum of cured and completed; cases regist'd, = the denominator for calculating treatment outcomes. The number of cases registered for treatment in 2006 is used as the denominator for calculating treatment outcomes unless it is less than the sum of outcomes, in which case the sum of outcomes is used. If the number of cases registered is not reported, then the number of cases notified in 2006 is used, or the sum of outcomes if the latter is greater. Data can be downloaded from http://stoptb.wpro.who.int.

| Smear-positive retreatment cases, DOTS | | | | | | | | | |
|---|---|---|---|---|---|---|---|---|---|
| | % of cohort | | | | | | | | |
| Number Regist'd | Cured | Com-pleted- | Died | Failed | Default | Trans-ferred | Not eval. | % Success | |
| | | | | | | | | | American Samoa |
| 55 | 7 | 69 | 5 | 0 | 4 | 4 | 11 | 76 | Australia |
| 12 | 75 | 25 | 0 | 0 | 0 | 0 | 0 | 100 | Brunei Darussalam |
| 711 | 77 | 6 | 6 | 4 | 2 | 5 | 0 | 83 | Cambodia |
| 70 163 | 84 | 5 | 2 | 2 | 1 | 5 | 0 | 89 | China |
| | | | | | | | | | Cook Islands |
| | | | | | | | | | Fiji |
| 4 | 50 | 0 | 50 | 0 | 0 | 0 | 0 | 50 | French Polynesia |
| 1 | 100 | 0 | 0 | 0 | 0 | 0 | 0 | 100 | Guam |
| 555 | 0 | 61 | 6 | 8 | 5 | 3 | 15 | 61 | Hong Kong (China) |
| 1423 | 14 | 24 | 13 | 1 | 9 | 2 | 38 | 38 | Japan |
| 5 | 100 | 0 | 0 | 0 | 0 | 0 | 0 | 100 | Kiribati |
| 149 | 83 | 3 | 7 | 5 | 3 | 0 | 0 | 86 | Lao People's Democratic Republic |
| 46 | 37 | 35 | 13 | 0 | 0 | 11 | 4 | 72 | Macao (China) |
| 1362 | 23 | 18 | 7 | 2 | 27 | 2 | 20 | 41 | Malaysia |
| 16 | 13 | 63 | 13 | 0 | 13 | 0 | 0 | 75 | Marshall Islands |
| 8 | 0 | 25 | 75 | 0 | 0 | 0 | 0 | 25 | Federated States of Micronesia |
| 609 | 43 | 33 | 6 | 12 | 5 | 1 | 0 | 76 | Mongolia |
| 1 | 100 | 0 | 0 | 0 | 0 | 0 | 0 | 100 | Nauru |
| 2 | 100 | 0 | 0 | 0 | 0 | 0 | 0 | 100 | New Caledonia |
| 17 | 0 | 65 | 24 | 0 | 0 | 6 | 6 | 65 | New Zealand |
| | | | | | | | | | Niue |
| 2 | 0 | 100 | 0 | 0 | 0 | 0 | 0 | 100 | Commonwealth of the Northern Mariana Islands |
| | | | | | | | | | Palau |
| | | | | | | | | | Papua New Guinea |
| 4101 | 53 | 18 | 4 | 6 | 7 | 4 | 7 | 72 | Philippines |
| 2698 | 70 | 2 | 1 | 1 | 6 | 20 | 0 | 72 | Republic of Korea |
| 1 | 100 | 0 | 0 | 0 | 0 | 0 | 0 | 100 | Samoa |
| 116 | 71 | 11 | 15 | 1 | 3 | 0 | 0 | 82 | Singapore |
| 9 | | 22 | 0 | 0 | 0 | 0 | 0 | 100 | Solomon Islands |
| | | | | | | | | | Tokelau |
| | | | | | | | | | Tonga |
| | | | | | | | | | Tuvalu |
| | | | | | | | | | Vanuatu |
| 7659 | 79 | 3 | 6 | 5 | 4 | 3 | 0 | 82 | Viet Nam |
| | | | | | | | | | Wallis and Futuna |
| **89 725** | **79** | **7** | **3** | **3** | **2** | **5** | **1** | **86** | **Western Pacific Region** |

**Table 51.** DOTS treatment success and case detection rates, 1994–2008

| | DOTS new smear-positive treatment success (%) | | | | | | | | | | | | | |
|---|---|---|---|---|---|---|---|---|---|---|---|---|---|---|
| | 1994 | 1995 | 1996 | 1997 | 1998 | 1999 | 2000 | 2001 | 2002 | 2003 | 2004 | 2005 | 2006 | 2007 |
| American Samoa | | 100 | | | 50 | 100 | 100 | 100 | 100 | 100 | 67 | 75 | | |
| Australia | | | | 66 | 75 | 84 | 74 | 66 | 78 | 82 | 85 | 80 | 85 | 85 |
| Brunei Darussalam | | | | | 85 | 76 | 63 | 56 | 84 | 60 | 71 | 71 | 84 | 76 |
| Cambodia | 84 | 91 | 94 | 91 | 95 | 93 | 91 | 92 | 92 | 93 | 91 | 93 | 93 | 94 |
| China | 94 | 96 | 96 | 96 | 97 | 96 | 95 | 96 | 93 | 94 | 94 | 94 | 94 | 94 |
| Cook Islands | 100 | 100 | 100 | 100 | | 67 | | | 100 | | | 100 | | 100 |
| Fiji | 90 | 86 | 86 | 91 | 90 | 92 | 85 | 85 | 78 | 86 | | 71 | 66 | 81 |
| French Polynesia | | 67 | 95 | 100 | 74 | 85 | 97 | 80 | 82 | 83 | 80 | 89 | 85 | 85 |
| Guam | | | | | | 94 | 93 | 71 | 68 | 96 | 100 | 85 | 90 | 89 |
| Hong Kong (China) | | | | | 85 | 78 | 76 | 78 | 79 | 78 | 80 | 77 | 78 | 66 |
| Japan | | | | | | 76 | 70 | 75 | 76 | 76 | 57 | 60 | 53 | 46 |
| Kiribati | | | | | 83 | 88 | 91 | 86 | 94 | 88 | 94 | 93 | 90 | 93 |
| Lao People's Democratic Republic | | 70 | 55 | 65 | 80 | 79 | 77 | 76 | 75 | 79 | 86 | 90 | 92 | 92 |
| Macao (China) | 75 | | | 81 | | 78 | 89 | 86 | 89 | 88 | 89 | 93 | 88 | 91 |
| Malaysia | | 69 | | | | 90 | 78 | 79 | 76 | 72 | 56 | 70 | 48 | 72 |
| Marshall Islands | | | | | 83 | 82 | 91 | 86 | 100 | 90 | 90 | 87 | 75 | 96 |
| Federated States of Micronesia | 64 | 80 | | | | 95 | 93 | 100 | 91 | 92 | 80 | 50 | 90 | 65 |
| Mongolia | | | 78 | 86 | 84 | 86 | 87 | 87 | 87 | 87 | 88 | 88 | 88 | 89 |
| Nauru | | | | | | 50 | 25 | 100 | 50 | | | 67 | 100 | 100 |
| New Caledonia | 62 | 75 | | | 70 | 77 | 89 | 84 | 85 | 75 | 94 | 94 | 89 | 77 |
| New Zealand | | | | | | | 30 | 9 | 60 | 36 | 68 | 60 | 70 | 86 |
| Niue | | | | | | | | | 100 | | | | | |
| Commonwealth of the Northern Mariana Islands | | | | | | 80 | 81 | 74 | 71 | 75 | 88 | 73 | 85 | 92 |
| Palau | 64 | 67 | 75 | | | | | 100 | 38 | 80 | 100 | 100 | 60 | |
| Papua New Guinea | | | | 93 | 72 | 66 | 63 | 67 | 53 | 58 | 65 | 71 | 73 | 39 |
| Philippines | 80 | | 82 | 83 | 84 | 87 | 88 | 88 | 88 | 88 | 87 | 89 | 88 | 89 |
| Republic of Korea | 71 | 76 | 71 | 82 | | | | | 83 | 82 | 80 | 83 | 81 | 82 |
| Samoa | 50 | 80 | 100 | | 86 | 94 | 92 | 77 | 84 | | 100 | 91 | | 92 |
| Singapore | 88 | 86 | | | | 95 | 85 | 88 | 87 | 77 | 81 | 83 | 84 | 81 |
| Solomon Islands | | 65 | 73 | 92 | 92 | | 81 | 89 | 90 | 87 | 87 | 85 | 90 | 92 |
| Tokelau | | | | | | | | | | | | | | |
| Tonga | 89 | 75 | 82 | 75 | 94 | 80 | 93 | 92 | 83 | | | 73 | 100 | 93 |
| Tuvalu | | | | | | | | | | | 100 | 100 | 75 | 75 |
| Vanuatu | | | | | | 88 | 88 | 88 | 79 | 75 | 90 | 81 | 90 | 93 |
| Viet Nam | 91 | 91 | 90 | 85 | 93 | 92 | 92 | 93 | 92 | 92 | 93 | 92 | 92 | 92 |
| Wallis and Futuna | | | | | | | | 100 | 100 | | 100 | | 100 | |
| **Western Pacific Region** | **90** | **91** | **93** | **93** | **95** | **94** | **92** | **93** | **90** | **91** | **91** | **92** | **92** | **92** |

Treatment success = sum of cured and completed; DOTS new smear-positive case detection rate = notified (new and relapse) cases divided by estimated incident cases. The table includes updated information; data shown here may differ from those published in previous reports. Data can be downloaded from http://stoptb.wpro.who.int.

| All forms case detection rate (%) | | | | | | | | | | | | | | |
|---|---|---|---|---|---|---|---|---|---|---|---|---|---|---|
| 1995 | 1996 | 1997 | 1998 | 1999 | 2000 | 2001 | 2002 | 2003 | 2004 | 2005 | 2006 | 2007 | 2008 | |
| | | 89 | 89 | 89 | 89 | 89 | 90 | 91 | 91 | 92 | 92 | 92 | 140 | American Samoa |
| 87 | | 87 | 87 | 87 | 87 | 87 | 87 | 87 | 87 | 87 | 87 | 87 | 87 | Australia |
| | | 87 | | 87 | 87 | 87 | 87 | 87 | 87 | 87 | 87 | 87 | 87 | Brunei Darussalam |
| 23 | 23 | 24 | 26 | 29 | 28 | 28 | 36 | 41 | 44 | 51 | 49 | 50 | 55 | Cambodia |
| 38 | 38 | 35 | 33 | 34 | 34 | 35 | 35 | 46 | 60 | 68 | 72 | 75 | 75 | China |
| 88 | 87 | 87 | | 84 | 82 | 79 | 76 | | 69 | 66 | 63 | | 50 | Cook Islands |
| 68 | 70 | 62 | 63 | 77 | 60 | 80 | 68 | 89 | 67 | 69 | 63 | 54 | 64 | Fiji |
| | 87 | 87 | 87 | 87 | 87 | 87 | 87 | 87 | 87 | 87 | 87 | 87 | 87 | French Polynesia |
| | | | | | 87 | 87 | 87 | 87 | 87 | 87 | 87 | 87 | 87 | Guam |
| 87 | 87 | 87 | 87 | 87 | 87 | 87 | 87 | 87 | 87 | 87 | 87 | 87 | 87 | Hong Kong (China) |
| 87 | 87 | 87 | 87 | 87 | 87 | 87 | 87 | 87 | 87 | 87 | 87 | 87 | 87 | Japan |
| | 92 | 130 | 78 | 72 | 71 | 54 | 56 | 81 | 88 | 95 | 110 | 96 | 97 | Kiribati |
| 10 | 17 | 23 | 25 | 28 | 25 | 27 | 30 | 31 | 35 | 42 | 43 | 42 | 44 | Lao People's Democratic Republic |
| 87 | 87 | 87 | 87 | | 87 | 87 | 87 | 87 | 87 | 87 | 87 | 87 | 87 | Macao (China) |
| 50 | 53 | 56 | 57 | 59 | 59 | 58 | 55 | 59 | 56 | 57 | 59 | 59 | 62 | Malaysia |
| | 43 | | 37 | 31 | 26 | 44 | 40 | 47 | 92 | 87 | 110 | 120 | 98 | Marshall Islands |
| 100 | 78 | 69 | 83 | | 67 | 79 | 100 | 81 | 99 | 85 | 94 | 130 | 160 | Federated States of Micronesia |
| 60 | 87 | 76 | 61 | 69 | 63 | 71 | 76 | 77 | 88 | 88 | 95 | 87 | 83 | Mongolia |
| | | | | 90 | 90 | 90 | 90 | 90 | | 90 | 90 | 90 | 420 | Nauru |
| 87 | 87 | 87 | 87 | 87 | 87 | 87 | 87 | 87 | 87 | 87 | 87 | 87 | 87 | New Caledonia |
| 87 | 87 | 87 | 87 | 87 | 87 | 87 | 87 | 87 | 87 | 87 | 87 | 87 | 87 | New Zealand |
| 0 | 95 | | | 91 | | | 88 | | | | | | | Niue |
| 87 | 87 | 87 | 87 | 87 | 87 | 87 | 87 | 87 | 87 | 87 | 87 | 87 | 87 | Commonwealth of the Northern Mariana Islands |
| 90 | 90 | 90 | | 90 | | | 90 | 90 | 90 | 90 | 90 | 90 | 0 | Palau |
| 68 | 26 | 64 | 89 | 99 | 78 | 92 | 79 | 88 | 86 | 82 | 81 | 94 | 85 | Papua New Guinea |
| 47 | 66 | 77 | 64 | 57 | 47 | 42 | 46 | 52 | 51 | 53 | 57 | 55 | 54 | Philippines |
| 87 | 87 | 87 | 87 | 87 | 87 | 87 | 87 | 87 | 87 | 87 | 87 | 87 | 87 | Republic of Korea |
| 98 | 69 | 73 | 51 | 73 | 100 | 55 | 79 | 71 | 92 | 57 | 72 | | 37 | Samoa |
| 87 | 87 | 87 | 87 | 87 | 87 | 87 | 87 | 87 | 87 | 87 | 87 | 87 | 87 | Singapore |
| 40 | 35 | 38 | 37 | 37 | 39 | 39 | 35 | 41 | 49 | 59 | 57 | 62 | 63 | Solomon Islands |
| 89 | | | | | | | | | | | | | | Tokelau |
| 67 | 75 | 73 | 110 | 79 | 88 | 45 | 110 | 61 | 46 | 71 | 72 | 93 | 53 | Tonga |
| 160 | | | 85 | 68 | 79 | 82 | 68 | 160 | | 69 | 53 | 110 | 110 | Tuvalu |
| 39 | 63 | 94 | 93 | 64 | 82 | 95 | 55 | 57 | 64 | 43 | 71 | 69 | 59 | Vanuatu |
| 37 | 49 | 51 | 56 | 56 | 56 | 56 | 56 | 56 | 56 | 56 | 56 | 56 | 56 | Viet Nam |
| 90 | 90 | 91 | | | | 91 | 91 | 91 | | 91 | | 91 | 0 | Wallis and Futuna |

**Table 52.** New smear-positive case notification by age and sex, absolute numbers, 2008

| | Male | | | | | | | Female | | | |
|---|---|---|---|---|---|---|---|---|---|---|---|
| | 0–14 | 15–24 | 25–34 | 35–44 | 45–54 | 55–64 | 65+ | 0–14 | 15–24 | 25–34 | 35–44 |
| American Samoa | | | | | | | | | | | |
| Australia | 2 | 46 | 33 | 20 | 27 | 23 | 42 | 3 | 27 | 32 | 14 |
| Brunei Darussalam | | 10 | 10 | 12 | 21 | 6 | 23 | 1 | 6 | 11 | 8 |
| Cambodia | 49 | 920 | 1570 | 2040 | 2117 | 1746 | 1683 | 72 | 808 | 1403 | 1809 |
| China | 751 | 45 596 | 44 651 | 56 182 | 55 740 | 57 492 | 69 678 | 964 | 29 223 | 23 484 | 22 370 |
| Cook Islands | | | | 1 | | 1 | | | | | |
| Fiji | | 10 | 10 | 4 | 9 | 4 | 4 | 13 | 6 | 5 | 6 |
| French Polynesia | 1 | 3 | 1 | 1 | 1 | 2 | 2 | | 1 | 1 | 1 |
| Guam | | | 1 | 7 | 8 | 3 | 4 | | 1 | 2 | |
| Hong Kong (China) | | 59 | 79 | 95 | 166 | 208 | 414 | 8 | 65 | 84 | 65 |
| Japan | 2 | 117 | 339 | 456 | 599 | 1063 | 3482 | 1 | 115 | 293 | 230 |
| Kiribati | 2 | 30 | 9 | 15 | 10 | 2 | 5 | 4 | 33 | 9 | 12 |
| Lao People's Democratic Republic | 6 | 159 | 262 | 329 | 380 | 409 | 373 | 10 | 101 | 165 | 209 |
| Macao (China) | 1 | 18 | 12 | 10 | 29 | 19 | 13 | 2 | 7 | 6 | 5 |
| Malaysia | 221 | 1436 | 2445 | 2318 | 2169 | 1599 | 1543 | 240 | 1161 | 1283 | 906 |
| Marshall Islands | 1 | 1 | 1 | 2 | 3 | | | 2 | 3 | 2 | 4 |
| Federated States of Micronesia | 1 | 9 | 3 | 1 | 3 | 1 | | 1 | 10 | 2 | 5 |
| Mongolia | 7 | 289 | 260 | 235 | 151 | 59 | 36 | 18 | 283 | 229 | 127 |
| Nauru | | 1 | | | 1 | | | | | | |
| New Caledonia | | 1 | 1 | | 2 | 1 | 2 | | | 1 | |
| New Zealand | | 9 | 4 | 9 | 5 | 10 | 18 | 1 | 8 | 13 | 9 |
| Niue | | | | | | | | | | | |
| Commonwealth of the Northern Mariana Islands | | 1 | | 1 | 5 | | 3 | | | | 2 |
| Palau | | | | | | | | | | | |
| Papua New Guinea | 65 | 250 | 207 | 160 | 95 | 58 | 12 | 74 | 261 | 230 | 113 |
| Philippines | 369 | 8735 | 11 741 | 13 529 | 12 808 | 8249 | 4348 | 341 | 4529 | 5452 | 5123 |
| Republic of Korea | 21 | 492 | 865 | 1093 | 1400 | 958 | 1848 | 32 | 483 | 722 | 483 |
| Samoa | | 1 | | | | 1 | | | 1 | 1 | 1 |
| Singapore | | 10 | 21 | 46 | 106 | 94 | 127 | | 9 | 16 | 20 |
| Solomon Islands | 3 | 17 | 12 | 11 | 10 | 11 | 7 | 4 | 13 | 23 | 11 |
| Tokelau | | | | | | | | | | | |
| Tonga | | 2 | | 2 | 2 | 1 | 1 | | | | |
| Tuvalu | 2 | 2 | 1 | | 1 | | | | 1 | 2 | 2 |
| Vanuatu | 1 | 4 | 4 | 3 | 5 | 4 | 3 | 4 | 3 | 4 | 1 |
| Viet Nam | 36 | 3401 | 7148 | 8230 | 8811 | 5158 | 6667 | 48 | 1993 | 2416 | 1820 |
| Wallis and Futuna | | | | | | | | | | | |
| **Western Pacific Region** | **1541** | **61 629** | **69 690** | **84 812** | **84 684** | **77 182** | **90 338** | **1843** | **39 151** | **35 891** | **33 356** |

| Female | | | All | | | | | | | Male/female ratio | |
|---|---|---|---|---|---|---|---|---|---|---|---|
| 45–54 | 55–64 | 65+ | 0–14 | 15–24 | 25–34 | 35–44 | 45–54 | 55–64 | 65+ | | |
| | | | | | | | | | | | American Samoa |
| 6 | 11 | 10 | 5 | 73 | 65 | 34 | 33 | 34 | 52 | 1.9 | Australia |
| 7 | 7 | 10 | 1 | 16 | 21 | 20 | 28 | 13 | 33 | 1.6 | Brunei Darussalam |
| 2093 | 1943 | 1607 | 121 | 1728 | 2973 | 3849 | 4210 | 3689 | 3290 | 1.0 | Cambodia |
| 17 565 | 17 814 | 21 086 | 1715 | 74 819 | 68 135 | 78 552 | 73 305 | 75 306 | 90 764 | 2.5 | China |
| | | | | | | 1 | | 1 | | | Cook Islands |
| 3 | 3 | 4 | 13 | 16 | 15 | 10 | 12 | 7 | 8 | 1.0 | Fiji |
| | 1 | 2 | 1 | 4 | 2 | 2 | 1 | 3 | 4 | 1.8 | French Polynesia |
| 1 | 1 | 3 | | 1 | 3 | 7 | 9 | 4 | 7 | 2.9 | Guam |
| 45 | 40 | 131 | 8 | 124 | 163 | 160 | 211 | 248 | 545 | 2.3 | Hong Kong (China) |
| 173 | 253 | 1872 | 3 | 232 | 632 | 686 | 772 | 1316 | 5354 | 2.1 | Japan |
| 9 | 3 | 4 | 6 | 63 | 18 | 27 | 19 | 5 | 9 | 1.0 | Kiribati |
| 264 | 220 | 192 | 16 | 260 | 427 | 538 | 644 | 629 | 565 | 1.7 | Lao People's Democratic Republic |
| 6 | 6 | 5 | 3 | 25 | 18 | 15 | 35 | 25 | 18 | 2.8 | Macao (China) |
| 878 | 648 | 657 | 461 | 2597 | 3728 | 3224 | 3047 | 2247 | 2200 | 2.0 | Malaysia |
| 5 | 1 | | 3 | 4 | 3 | 6 | 8 | 1 | | 0.5 | Marshall Islands |
| 1 | | | 2 | 19 | 5 | 6 | 4 | 1 | | 0.9 | Federated States of Micronesia |
| 86 | 32 | 26 | 25 | 572 | 489 | 362 | 237 | 91 | 62 | 1.3 | Mongolia |
| | | | | 1 | | | 1 | | | | Nauru |
| | | 1 | | 1 | 2 | | 2 | 1 | 3 | 3.5 | New Caledonia |
| 3 | 3 | 9 | 1 | 17 | 17 | 18 | 8 | 13 | 27 | 1.2 | New Zealand |
| | | | | | | | | | | | Niue |
| | 1 | | | 1 | | 3 | 5 | 1 | 3 | 3.3 | Commonwealth of the Northern Mariana Islands |
| | | | | | | | | | | | Palau |
| 75 | 48 | 10 | 139 | 511 | 437 | 273 | 170 | 106 | 22 | 1.0 | Papua New Guinea |
| 4527 | 3086 | 2188 | 710 | 13 264 | 17 193 | 18 652 | 17 335 | 11 335 | 6536 | 2.4 | Philippines |
| 402 | 360 | 1889 | 53 | 975 | 1587 | 1576 | 1802 | 1318 | 3737 | 1.5 | Republic of Korea |
| | | 1 | | 2 | 1 | 1 | | 1 | 1 | 0.5 | Samoa |
| 26 | 17 | 33 | | 19 | 37 | 66 | 132 | 111 | 160 | 3.3 | Singapore |
| 13 | 3 | 2 | 7 | 30 | 35 | 22 | 23 | 14 | 9 | 1.0 | Solomon Islands |
| | | | | | | | | | | | Tokelau |
| 1 | 2 | | | 2 | | 2 | 3 | 3 | 1 | 2.7 | Tonga |
| 1 | | | 2 | 3 | 3 | 2 | 2 | | | 1.0 | Tuvalu |
| 3 | 5 | 1 | 5 | 7 | 8 | 4 | 8 | 9 | 4 | 1.1 | Vanuatu |
| 2087 | 1858 | 3811 | 84 | 5394 | 9564 | 10 050 | 10 898 | 7016 | 10 478 | 2.8 | Viet Nam |
| | | | | | | | | | | | Wallis and Futuna |
| **28 280** | **26 366** | **33 554** | **3384** | **100 780** | **105 581** | **118 168** | **112 964** | **103 548** | **123 892** | **2.4** | **Western Pacific Region** |

**Table 53.** New smear-positive case notification rates per 100 000 population by age and sex, 2008

| | Male | | | | | | | Female | | | |
|---|---|---|---|---|---|---|---|---|---|---|---|
| | 0–14 | 15–24 | 25–34 | 35–44 | 45–54 | 55–64 | 65+ | 0–14 | 15–24 | 25–34 | 35–44 |
| American Samoa | | | | | | | | | | | |
| Australia | 0 | 3 | 2 | 1 | 2 | 2 | 4 | 0 | 2 | 2 | 1 |
| Brunei Darussalam | 0 | 29 | 28 | 43 | 95 | 60 | 383 | 2 | 19 | 29 | 30 |
| Cambodia | 2 | 56 | 181 | 286 | 457 | 649 | 1130 | 3 | 50 | 157 | 220 |
| China | 0 | 40 | 40 | 48 | 66 | 109 | 145 | 1 | 28 | 22 | 20 |
| Cook Islands | | | | | | | | | | | |
| Fiji | 0 | 12 | 16 | 8 | 21 | 15 | 29 | 10 | 8 | 9 | 12 |
| French Polynesia | 3 | 12 | 5 | 5 | 7 | 22 | 29 | 0 | 4 | 5 | 5 |
| Guam | 0 | 0 | 8 | 54 | 89 | 50 | 80 | 0 | 8 | 17 | 0 |
| Hong Kong (China) | 0 | 13 | 16 | 16 | 29 | 63 | 105 | 2 | 15 | 14 | 9 |
| Japan | 0 | 2 | 4 | 5 | 7 | 12 | 33 | 0 | 2 | 3 | 3 |
| Kiribati | | | | | | | | | | | |
| Lao People's Democratic Republic | 1 | 26 | 64 | 118 | 196 | 449 | 429 | 1 | 17 | 39 | 71 |
| Macao (China) | 3 | 46 | 41 | 26 | 66 | 90 | 87 | 5 | 17 | 16 | 10 |
| Malaysia | 5 | 58 | 120 | 131 | 162 | 212 | 297 | 6 | 48 | 65 | 53 |
| Marshall Islands | | | | | | | | | | | |
| Federated States of Micronesia | 5 | 69 | 43 | 17 | 75 | 50 | 0 | 5 | 83 | 29 | 83 |
| Mongolia | 2 | 97 | 112 | 131 | 147 | 113 | 86 | 5 | 97 | 99 | 69 |
| Nauru | | | | | | | | | | | |
| New Caledonia | 0 | 5 | 6 | 0 | 15 | 11 | 29 | 0 | 0 | 5 | 0 |
| New Zealand | 0 | 3 | 1 | 3 | 2 | 5 | 8 | 0 | 3 | 5 | 3 |
| Niue | | | | | | | | | | | |
| Commonwealth of the Northern Mariana Islands | | | | | | | | | | | |
| Palau | | | | | | | | | | | |
| Papua New Guinea | 5 | 42 | 45 | 46 | 44 | 50 | 17 | 6 | 45 | 49 | 32 |
| Philippines | 2 | 102 | 177 | 278 | 376 | 407 | 303 | 2 | 55 | 84 | 105 |
| Republic of Korea | 0 | 14 | 21 | 26 | 41 | 44 | 100 | 1 | 14 | 18 | 12 |
| Samoa | 0 | 6 | 0 | 0 | 0 | 25 | 0 | 0 | 7 | 9 | 9 |
| Singapore | 0 | 3 | 7 | 12 | 28 | 44 | 76 | 0 | 3 | 6 | 5 |
| Solomon Islands | 3 | 34 | 31 | 48 | 67 | 122 | 100 | 4 | 28 | 64 | 46 |
| Tokelau | | | | | | | | | | | |
| Tonga | 0 | 17 | 0 | 40 | 67 | 50 | 33 | 0 | 0 | 0 | 0 |
| Tuvalu | | | | | | | | | | | |
| Vanuatu | 2 | 18 | 27 | 27 | 63 | 80 | 75 | 10 | 14 | 25 | 8 |
| Viet Nam | 0 | 38 | 100 | 144 | 229 | 276 | 303 | 0 | 23 | 34 | 31 |
| Wallis and Futuna | | | | | | | | | | | |
| **Western Pacific Region** | **1** | **41** | **48** | **58** | **78** | **108** | **135** | **1** | **28** | **26** | **24** |

Rates are per 100 000 population of each age/sex group. Rates are calculated excluding those countries for which breakdown of notified cases or population by age and sex is missing.
Data can be downloaded from http://stoptb.wpro.who.int.

| Female | | | All | | | | | | | |
|---|---|---|---|---|---|---|---|---|---|---|
| 45–54 | 55–64 | 65+ | 0–14 | 15–24 | 25–34 | 35–44 | 45–54 | 55–64 | 65+ | |
| | | | | | | | | | | American Samoa |
| 0 | 1 | 1 | 0 | 3 | 2 | 1 | 1 | 2 | 2 | Australia |
| 41 | 117 | 167 | 1 | 24 | 28 | 36 | 72 | 81 | 275 | Brunei Darussalam |
| 358 | 506 | 562 | 2 | 53 | 169 | 250 | 402 | 565 | 756 | Cambodia |
| 22 | 36 | 40 | 1 | 34 | 32 | 34 | 45 | 73 | 90 | China |
| | | | | | | | | | | Cook Islands |
| 7 | 11 | 21 | 5 | 10 | 13 | 10 | 14 | 13 | 24 | Fiji |
| 0 | 13 | 29 | 1 | 8 | 5 | 5 | 4 | 18 | 29 | French Polynesia |
| 11 | 17 | 50 | 0 | 4 | 13 | 28 | 50 | 33 | 64 | Guam |
| 7 | 13 | 29 | 1 | 14 | 15 | 12 | 18 | 39 | 64 | Hong Kong (China) |
| 2 | 3 | 13 | 0 | 2 | 3 | 4 | 5 | 7 | 21 | Japan |
| | | | | | | | | | | Kiribati |
| 131 | 208 | 175 | 1 | 21 | 52 | 94 | 163 | 319 | 287 | Lao People's Democratic Republic |
| 14 | 35 | 24 | 4 | 31 | 27 | 17 | 41 | 66 | 50 | Macao (China) |
| 69 | 91 | 110 | 6 | 53 | 93 | 93 | 116 | 153 | 197 | Malaysia |
| | | | | | | | | | | Marshall Islands |
| 25 | 0 | 0 | 5 | 76 | 36 | 50 | 50 | 25 | 0 | Federated States of Micronesia |
| 80 | 58 | 46 | 3 | 97 | 105 | 100 | 112 | 85 | 63 | Mongolia |
| | | | | | | | | | | Nauru |
| 0 | 0 | 11 | 0 | 3 | 5 | 0 | 8 | 6 | 19 | New Caledonia |
| 1 | 1 | 3 | 0 | 3 | 3 | 3 | 1 | 3 | 5 | New Zealand |
| | | | | | | | | | | Niue |
| | | | | | | | | | | Commonwealth of the Northern Mariana Islands |
| | | | | | | | | | | Palau |
| 35 | 43 | 14 | 6 | 43 | 47 | 39 | 39 | 46 | 15 | Papua New Guinea |
| 130 | 147 | 122 | 2 | 79 | 131 | 192 | 251 | 275 | 202 | Philippines |
| 12 | 16 | 71 | 1 | 14 | 20 | 19 | 26 | 30 | 83 | Republic of Korea |
| 0 | 0 | 20 | 0 | 6 | 4 | 4 | 0 | 13 | 11 | Samoa |
| 7 | 8 | 17 | 0 | 3 | 6 | 8 | 18 | 25 | 43 | Singapore |
| 93 | 33 | 29 | 4 | 31 | 47 | 47 | 79 | 78 | 64 | Solomon Islands |
| | | | | | | | | | | Tokelau |
| 25 | 67 | 0 | 0 | 9 | 0 | 20 | 43 | 60 | 17 | Tonga |
| | | | | | | | | | | Tuvalu |
| 43 | 100 | 33 | 6 | 16 | 26 | 17 | 53 | 90 | 57 | Vanuatu |
| 53 | 94 | 151 | 0 | 31 | 67 | 87 | 139 | 183 | 222 | Viet Nam |
| | | | | | | | | | | Wallis and Futuna |
| **27** | **38** | **43** | **1** | **35** | **37** | **41** | **53** | **74** | **86** | **Western Pacific Region** |

**Table 54.** Number of TB cases notified, 1980–2008

| | 1980 | 1981 | 1982 | 1983 | 1984 | 1985 | 1986 | 1987 | 1988 | 1989 | 1990 | 1991 | 1992 | 1993 |
|---|---|---|---|---|---|---|---|---|---|---|---|---|---|---|
| American Samoa | 2 | 6 | 6 | 8 | 12 | 5 | 8 | 9 | 13 | 5 | 9 | 3 | 1 | 4 |
| Australia | 1457 | 1386 | 1270 | 1219 | 1299 | 1088 | 906 | 907 | 954 | 952 | 1016 | 950 | 1011 | 991 |
| Brunei Darussalam | 196 | 285 | 245 | 276 | 256 | 238 | 212 | 189 | 126 | 128 | 143 | | 180 | 160 |
| Cambodia | 2576 | 1980 | 8158 | 7572 | 10 241 | 10 145 | 10 325 | 9106 | 10 691 | 7906 | 6501 | 10 903 | 16 148 | 13 270 |
| China | | | 98 654 | 117 557 | 151 564 | 226 899 | 265 095 | 251 600 | 304 639 | 310 607 | 375 481 | 345 000 | 320 426 | 344 218 |
| Cook Islands | 8 | 2 | 12 | 15 | 3 | 8 | 3 | 2 | | 2 | | 1 | 6 | 5 |
| Fiji | 210 | 180 | 163 | 185 | 165 | 230 | 199 | 173 | 162 | 218 | 226 | 247 | 240 | 183 |
| French Polynesia | 76 | 66 | 65 | 78 | 80 | 78 | 85 | 80 | 63 | 73 | 59 | 49 | 83 | 78 |
| Guam | 55 | 41 | 49 | 48 | 54 | 37 | 49 | 34 | 41 | 75 | | | 60 | 70 |
| Hong Kong (China) | 8065 | 7729 | 7527 | 7301 | 7843 | 7545 | 7432 | 7269 | 7021 | 6704 | 6510 | 6283 | 6534 | 6537 |
| Japan | 70 916 | 65 867 | 63 940 | 62 021 | 61 521 | 58 567 | 56 690 | 56 496 | 54 357 | 53 112 | 51 821 | 50 612 | 48 956 | 48 461 |
| Kiribati | 146 | 187 | 193 | 127 | 111 | 103 | 129 | 110 | 208 | 121 | 68 | 91 | 100 | 99 |
| Lao People's Democratic Republic | 7630 | | 4706 | 4700 | 6528 | 4258 | 1514 | 3468 | 7279 | 2952 | 1826 | 1951 | 994 | 2093 |
| Macao (China) | 1101 | 585 | 233 | 455 | 671 | 571 | 420 | 389 | 320 | 274 | 343 | 329 | 294 | 285 |
| Malaysia | 11 218 | 10 970 | 11 944 | 11 634 | 10 577 | 10 569 | 10 735 | 11 068 | 10 944 | 10 686 | 11 702 | 11 059 | 11 420 | 12 285 |
| Marshall Islands | 6 | 7 | 12 | 15 | 12 | 15 | 37 | 32 | 11 | 7 | | 26 | 52 | 61 |
| Federated States of Micronesia | | | 67 | 73 | 75 | 66 | 60 | 98 | 77 | 68 | 367 | 350 | 111 | 151 |
| Mongolia | 1160 | 1094 | 1325 | 1514 | 1652 | 2994 | 2819 | 2433 | 2538 | 2233 | 1659 | 1611 | 1516 | 1418 |
| Nauru | | 2 | 8 | | | | 8 | 6 | 8 | | 7 | | | |
| New Caledonia | 108 | 128 | 120 | 171 | 144 | 104 | 98 | 74 | 111 | 128 | 143 | 140 | 140 | 104 |
| New Zealand | 474 | 448 | 437 | 415 | 404 | 359 | 320 | 296 | 295 | 303 | 348 | 335 | 317 | 274 |
| Niue | 1 | | 2 | 3 | 1 | | 5 | | 3 | | | | 2 | 1 |
| Commonwealth of the Northern Mariana Islands | | 26 | 75 | 74 | 58 | 64 | 16 | 56 | 27 | 28 | 28 | | 67 | |
| Palau | 17 | 10 | 17 | 14 | 20 | 26 | 13 | 38 | 17 | 3 | | 6 | 4 | 25 |
| Papua New Guinea | 2525 | 2508 | 2742 | 2955 | 3505 | 3453 | 2877 | 2251 | 4261 | 3396 | 2497 | 3401 | 2540 | 7451 |
| Philippines | 112 307 | 116 821 | 104 715 | 106 300 | 151 863 | 151 028 | 153 129 | 163 740 | 183 113 | 217 272 | 317 008 | 207 371 | 236 172 | 178 134 |
| Republic of Korea | 89 803 | 98 532 | 100 878 | 91 572 | 85 669 | 87 169 | 88 789 | 87 419 | 74 460 | 70 012 | 63 904 | 57 864 | 48 070 | 46 999 |
| Samoa | 59 | 49 | 43 | 41 | 37 | 43 | 65 | 29 | 29 | 37 | 44 | 44 | 26 | 49 |
| Singapore | 2710 | 2425 | 2179 | 2065 | 2143 | 1952 | 1760 | 1616 | 1666 | 1617 | 1591 | 1841 | 1778 | 1830 |
| Solomon Islands | 266 | 313 | 324 | 302 | 337 | 377 | 292 | 334 | 372 | 488 | 382 | 309 | 364 | 367 |
| Tokelau | | 1 | | | | 2 | | 9 | 1 | | 1 | 1 | 1 | |
| Tonga | 64 | 49 | 45 | 50 | 54 | 49 | 35 | 24 | 14 | 36 | 23 | 20 | 29 | 33 |
| Tuvalu | 33 | 18 | 12 | 23 | 9 | 32 | 27 | 22 | 24 | 26 | 23 | 30 | 30 | 28 |
| Vanuatu | 178 | 92 | 173 | 196 | 188 | 124 | 131 | 90 | 118 | 144 | 140 | 230 | 193 | 114 |
| Viet Nam | 43 062 | 43 506 | 51 206 | 43 185 | 43 875 | 46 941 | 47 557 | 55 505 | 52 463 | 52 270 | 50 203 | 59 784 | 56 594 | 52 994 |
| Wallis and Futuna | 23 | 24 | 5 | 17 | 14 | 14 | | 34 | 1 | 30 | | 22 | 4 | 11 |
| **Western Pacific Region** | **356 452** | **355 337** | **461 550** | **462 181** | **540 985** | **615 153** | **651 840** | **655 006** | **716 427** | **741 913** | **894 073** | **760 863** | **754 463** | **718 783** |
| Number reporting | 36 | 33 | 36 | 36 | 36 | 36 | 35 | 36 | 36 | 35 | 32 | 31 | 35 | 33 |
| % reporting | 100 | 92 | 100 | 100 | 100 | 100 | 97 | 100 | 100 | 97 | 89 | 86 | 97 | 92 |

From 1995, number shown is all notified new and relapse cases (DOTS and non-DOTS). The table includes updated information; data shown here may differ from those published in previous reports. Data can be downloaded from http://stoptb.wpro.who.int.

| 1994 | 1995 | 1996 | 1997 | 1998 | 1999 | 2000 | 2001 | 2002 | 2003 | 2004 | 2005 | 2006 | 2007 | 2008 | |
|---|---|---|---|---|---|---|---|---|---|---|---|---|---|---|---|
| 4 | | | 6 | 3 | 4 | 3 | 3 | 2 | 3 | 5 | 6 | 4 | 3 | 3 | American Samoa |
| 1057 | 1073 | | 1145 | 899 | 1073 | 1043 | 980 | 1013 | 949 | 1059 | 1046 | 1159 | 1115 | 1213 | Australia |
| | | | 160 | | 272 | 307 | 216 | 230 | 206 | 176 | 163 | 202 | 207 | 223 | Brunei Darussalam |
| 15 172 | 14 603 | 14 857 | 15 629 | 16 946 | 19 266 | 18 891 | 19 170 | 24 610 | 28 216 | 30 838 | 35 535 | 34 660 | 35 601 | 38 927 | Cambodia |
| 363 804 | 515 764 | 504 758 | 466 394 | 445 704 | 449 518 | 454 372 | 470 221 | 462 609 | 615 868 | 790 603 | 834 428 | 940 889 | 979 502 | 975 821 | China |
| 4 | 2 | 1 | 2 | | 3 | 1 | 2 | 1 | | 1 | 1 | 1 | | 2 | Cook Islands |
| 225 | 203 | 200 | 171 | 166 | 192 | 144 | 183 | 148 | 185 | 134 | 132 | 114 | 94 | 106 | Fiji |
| 89 | | 86 | 91 | 105 | 93 | 62 | 62 | 64 | 50 | 60 | 63 | 69 | 64 | 50 | French Polynesia |
| 94 | | | | | | 54 | 63 | 51 | 22 | 50 | 63 | 44 | 53 | 89 | Guam |
| 6319 | 6212 | 6501 | 7072 | 7673 | 5605 | 6015 | 6788 | 6277 | 5914 | 5684 | 5660 | 5356 | 5363 | 5544 | Hong Kong (China) |
| 44 425 | 43 078 | 42 122 | 42 190 | 44 016 | 40 800 | 39 384 | 35 489 | 32 828 | 31 638 | 29 736 | 27 194 | 25 304 | 24 779 | 24 181 | Japan |
| 253 | | 327 | 464 | 276 | 255 | 252 | 189 | 196 | 284 | 310 | 332 | 378 | 334 | 335 | Kiribati |
| 1135 | 830 | 1440 | 1923 | 2149 | 2420 | 2227 | 2418 | 2621 | 2748 | 3162 | 3777 | 3958 | 3905 | 4048 | Lao People's Democratic Republic |
| | 402 | 570 | 575 | 465 | | 449 | 465 | 388 | 371 | 309 | 355 | 374 | 342 | 359 | Macao (China) |
| 11 708 | 11 778 | 12 691 | 13 539 | 14 115 | 14 908 | 15 057 | 14 830 | 14 389 | 15 671 | 14 986 | 15 342 | 16 051 | 16 129 | 17 144 | Malaysia |
| | | 59 | | 49 | 41 | 34 | 56 | 51 | 60 | 117 | 111 | 138 | 158 | 125 | Marshall Islands |
| 173 | 172 | 126 | 107 | 123 | | 91 | 104 | 127 | 99 | 118 | 98 | 104 | 137 | 164 | Federated States of Micronesia |
| 1730 | 2780 | 4062 | 3592 | 2915 | 3348 | 3109 | 3526 | 3829 | 3918 | 4542 | 4601 | 5049 | 4654 | 4490 | Mongolia |
| 4 | | | | | 2 | 4 | 3 | 5 | 3 | | 11 | 12 | 3 | 5 | Nauru |
| 97 | 87 | 104 | 88 | 90 | 78 | 94 | 61 | 65 | 38 | 61 | 47 | 48 | 47 | 44 | New Caledonia |
| 352 | 391 | 352 | 321 | 365 | 447 | 344 | 377 | 329 | 386 | 371 | 332 | 344 | 274 | 292 | New Zealand |
| 2 | | 2 | | | 1 | | | 4 | | | | | | 0 | Niue |
| 46 | 48 | 51 | 93 | 97 | 66 | 75 | 58 | 53 | 45 | 53 | 57 | 51 | 44 | 28 | Commonwealth of the Northern Mariana Islands |
| 41 | 19 | 5 | 15 | | 32 | | | 11 | 9 | 5 | 10 | 12 | 11 | | Palau |
| 5335 | 8041 | 3195 | 7977 | 11 291 | 13 003 | 10 520 | 12 658 | 11 197 | 12 798 | 12 743 | 12 564 | 12 620 | 15 002 | 13 984 | Papua New Guinea |
| 180 044 | 119 186 | 165 453 | 195 767 | 162 360 | 145 807 | 119 914 | 107 133 | 118 408 | 132 759 | 130 530 | 137 100 | 147 305 | 140 588 | 139 603 | Philippines |
| 38 155 | 42 117 | 39 315 | 33 215 | 34 661 | 32 075 | 21 782 | 37 268 | 34 967 | 33 843 | 34 389 | 38 290 | 37 861 | 37 554 | 36 847 | Republic of Korea |
| 45 | 45 | 31 | 32 | 22 | 31 | 43 | 22 | 31 | 27 | 34 | 24 | 25 | | 12 | Samoa |
| 1677 | 1889 | 1951 | 1977 | 2120 | 1805 | 1728 | 1536 | 1516 | 1581 | 1414 | 1356 | 1314 | 1359 | 1549 | Singapore |
| 332 | 352 | 299 | 318 | 295 | 289 | 302 | 292 | 256 | 293 | 340 | 397 | 371 | 397 | 387 | Solomon Islands |
| | 2 | | | | | | | | | | | | | 0 | Tokelau |
| 23 | 20 | 22 | 21 | 30 | 22 | 24 | 12 | 29 | 16 | 12 | 18 | 18 | 23 | 13 | Tonga |
| 19 | 36 | | | 18 | 14 | 16 | 16 | 13 | 30 | | 12 | 9 | 18 | 17 | Tuvalu |
| 152 | 79 | 126 | 184 | 178 | 120 | 152 | 175 | 101 | 104 | 115 | 76 | 126 | 122 | 103 | Vanuatu |
| 51 763 | 55 739 | 74 711 | 77 838 | 87 468 | 88 879 | 89 792 | 90 728 | 95 044 | 92 741 | 98 173 | 94 916 | 97 363 | 97 400 | 97 772 | Viet Nam |
| 11 | 6 | 8 | 14 | | | | 1 | 19 | 15 | | 7 | | 2 | | Wallis and Futuna |
| 724 290 | 824 954 | 873 425 | 870 920 | 834 599 | 820 469 | 786 285 | 805 105 | 811 482 | 980 890 | 1 160 130 | 1 274 124 | 1 331 333 | 1 365 284 | 1 363 480 | **Western Pacific Region** |
| 33 | 29 | 31 | 31 | 30 | 32 | 34 | 35 | 35 | 36 | 32 | 35 | 35 | 34 | 34 | Number reporting |
| 92 | 81 | 86 | 86 | 83 | 89 | 94 | 97 | 97 | 100 | 89 | 100 | 97 | 94 | 94 | % reporting |

**Table 55.** Case notification rates, 1980–2008

| | 1980 | 1981 | 1982 | 1983 | 1984 | 1985 | 1986 | 1987 | 1988 | 1989 | 1990 | 1991 | 1992 | 1993 |
|---|---|---|---|---|---|---|---|---|---|---|---|---|---|---|
| American Samoa | 6 | 18 | 17 | 22 | 32 | 13 | 19 | 21 | 29 | 11 | 19 | 6 | 2 | 8 |
| Australia | 10 | 9 | 8 | 8 | 8 | 7 | 6 | 6 | 6 | 6 | 6 | 6 | 6 | 6 |
| Brunei Darussalam | 102 | 143 | 120 | 131 | 118 | 107 | 92 | 80 | 52 | 51 | 56 | | 66 | 57 |
| Cambodia | 38 | 29 | 114 | 102 | 132 | 125 | 123 | 104 | 118 | 84 | 67 | 109 | 155 | 124 |
| China | | | 10 | 11 | 14 | 21 | 24 | 23 | 27 | 27 | 33 | 30 | 27 | 29 |
| Cook Islands | 45 | 11 | 68 | 85 | 17 | 45 | 17 | 11 | 0 | 11 | 0 | 6 | 33 | 28 |
| Fiji | 33 | 28 | 24 | 27 | 24 | 32 | 28 | 24 | 23 | 30 | 31 | 34 | 32 | 24 |
| French Polynesia | 50 | 42 | 41 | 47 | 47 | 45 | 48 | 44 | 34 | 38 | 30 | 25 | 41 | 38 |
| Guam | 52 | 38 | 44 | 42 | 46 | 31 | 40 | 27 | 32 | 57 | | | 43 | 50 |
| Hong Kong (China) | 160 | 150 | 144 | 137 | 145 | 138 | 135 | 131 | 126 | 119 | 114 | 109 | 111 | 109 |
| Japan | 61 | 56 | 54 | 52 | 51 | 48 | 47 | 46 | 44 | 43 | 42 | 41 | 39 | 39 |
| Kiribati | 267 | 333 | 335 | 214 | 182 | 164 | 200 | 166 | 304 | 172 | 95 | 124 | 135 | 132 |
| Lao People's Democratic Republic | 246 | | 145 | 141 | 191 | 121 | 42 | 93 | 190 | 75 | 45 | 46 | 23 | 47 |
| Macao (China) | 437 | 226 | 87 | 163 | 229 | 186 | 131 | 117 | 92 | 76 | 92 | 86 | 75 | 72 |
| Malaysia | 82 | 78 | 83 | 78 | 69 | 67 | 67 | 67 | 64 | 61 | 65 | 59 | 60 | 63 |
| Marshall Islands | 20 | 22 | 36 | 43 | 33 | 39 | 92 | 76 | 25 | 15 | | 54 | 105 | 122 |
| Federated States of Micronesia | | | 86 | 91 | 90 | 77 | 68 | 109 | 84 | 72 | 381 | 354 | 110 | 146 |
| Mongolia | 70 | 64 | 76 | 84 | 89 | 157 | 143 | 120 | 121 | 103 | 75 | 71 | 66 | 61 |
| Nauru | 0 | 26 | 104 | 0 | 0 | 0 | 96 | 70 | 91 | 0 | 77 | | | |
| New Caledonia | 76 | 88 | 81 | 114 | 94 | 67 | 62 | 46 | 68 | 76 | 84 | 80 | 78 | 57 |
| New Zealand | 15 | 14 | 14 | 13 | 13 | 11 | 10 | 9 | 9 | 9 | 10 | 10 | 9 | 8 |
| Niue | 29 | 0 | 64 | 100 | 35 | 0 | 190 | 0 | 125 | | 0 | | 89 | 44 |
| Commonwealth of the Northern Mariana Islands | | 139 | 355 | 308 | 214 | 213 | 49 | 157 | 70 | 68 | 64 | | 135 | |
| Palau | 139 | 80 | 134 | 108 | 150 | 191 | 94 | 269 | 118 | 21 | | 39 | 25 | 155 |
| Papua New Guinea | 79 | 77 | 82 | 86 | 99 | 95 | 77 | 59 | 109 | 84 | 60 | 80 | 58 | 167 |
| Philippines | 234 | 237 | 207 | 205 | 286 | 278 | 275 | 287 | 314 | 363 | 518 | 331 | 368 | 272 |
| Republic of Korea | 236 | 255 | 257 | 230 | 212 | 214 | 215 | 210 | 177 | 165 | 149 | 134 | 110 | 106 |
| Samoa | 38 | 32 | 28 | 26 | 24 | 27 | 41 | 18 | 18 | 23 | 27 | 27 | 16 | 30 |
| Singapore | 112 | 98 | 86 | 80 | 81 | 72 | 64 | 57 | 58 | 55 | 53 | 59 | 56 | 56 |
| Solomon Islands | 116 | 132 | 132 | 119 | 128 | 139 | 104 | 116 | 125 | 160 | 122 | 96 | 110 | 107 |
| Tokelau | 0 | 64 | 0 | 0 | 0 | 126 | 0 | 559 | 62 | 0 | 62 | 63 | 64 | |
| Tonga | 66 | 51 | 47 | 53 | 58 | 53 | 38 | 26 | 15 | 38 | 24 | 21 | 30 | 34 |
| Tuvalu | 410 | 221 | 145 | 274 | 106 | 370 | 307 | 245 | 263 | 280 | 244 | 315 | 312 | 289 |
| Vanuatu | 152 | 77 | 141 | 156 | 146 | 94 | 97 | 65 | 83 | 99 | 94 | 150 | 122 | 70 |
| Viet Nam | 81 | 80 | 93 | 76 | 76 | 79 | 79 | 90 | 83 | 81 | 76 | 88 | 82 | 75 |
| Wallis and Futuna | 200 | 200 | 40 | 130 | 104 | 101 | | 243 | 7 | 216 | | 158 | 29 | 78 |
| **Western Pacific Region** | **27** | **27** | **34** | **34** | **39** | **44** | **46** | **45** | **49** | **50** | **59** | **50** | **49** | **46** |

Rates are per 100 000 population. The table includes updated information; data shown here may differ from those published in previous reports. Data can be downloaded from http://stoptb.wpro.who.int.

| 1994 | 1995 | 1996 | 1997 | 1998 | 1999 | 2000 | 2001 | 2002 | 2003 | 2004 | 2005 | 2006 | 2007 | 2008 | |
|---|---|---|---|---|---|---|---|---|---|---|---|---|---|---|---|
| 8 | | 0 | 11 | 5 | 7 | 5 | 5 | 3 | 5 | 8 | 9 | 5 | 4 | 5 | American Samoa |
| 6 | 6 | | 6 | 5 | 6 | 5 | 5 | 5 | 5 | 5 | 5 | 5 | 5 | 6 | Australia |
| | | | 52 | | 84 | 92 | 63 | 66 | 58 | 48 | 44 | 53 | 53 | 55 | Brunei Darussalam |
| 137 | 128 | 127 | 130 | 138 | 154 | 148 | 147 | 186 | 209 | 225 | 255 | 244 | 246 | 267 | Cambodia |
| 30 | 42 | 41 | 38 | 36 | 36 | 36 | 37 | 36 | 47 | 61 | 68 | 71 | 74 | 73 | China |
| 22 | 11 | 6 | 11 | 0 | 18 | 6 | 13 | 7 | 0 | 7 | 7 | 7 | | 10 | Cook Islands |
| 30 | 26 | 26 | 22 | 21 | 24 | 18 | 23 | 18 | 23 | 16 | 16 | 14 | 11 | 13 | Fiji |
| 42 | | 39 | 41 | 46 | 40 | 26 | 26 | 26 | 20 | 24 | 25 | 27 | 24 | 19 | French Polynesia |
| 66 | | | | | | 35 | 40 | 32 | 13 | 30 | 37 | 26 | 31 | 51 | Guam |
| 104 | 100 | 103 | 111 | 118 | 85 | 90 | 101 | 92 | 86 | 81 | 80 | 75 | 74 | 79 | Hong Kong (China) |
| 36 | 34 | 33 | 33 | 35 | 32 | 31 | 28 | 26 | 25 | 23 | 21 | 20 | 19 | 19 | Japan |
| 332 | | 417 | 582 | 340 | 309 | 300 | 221 | 225 | 320 | 343 | 361 | 404 | 351 | 304 | Kiribati |
| 25 | 18 | 30 | 39 | 43 | 47 | 43 | 45 | 49 | 50 | 57 | 67 | 69 | 67 | 69 | Lao People's Democratic Republic |
| | 98 | 136 | 136 | 108 | | 102 | 104 | 85 | 80 | 66 | 75 | 78 | 71 | 75 | Macao (China) |
| 58 | 57 | 60 | 62 | 64 | 66 | 65 | 62 | 59 | 63 | 59 | 60 | 51 | 61 | 65 | Malaysia |
| | | 115 | | 95 | 79 | 65 | 106 | 95 | 110 | 211 | 196 | 238 | 267 | 206 | Marshall Islands |
| 163 | 160 | 117 | 99 | 114 | | 85 | 97 | 118 | 91 | 108 | 89 | 94 | 123 | 165 | Federated States of Micronesia |
| 73 | 116 | 169 | 148 | 119 | 136 | 126 | 142 | 153 | 155 | 178 | 173 | 194 | 177 | 170 | Mongolia |
| 41 | | | | | 20 | 40 | 30 | 50 | 30 | | 109 | 118 | 30 | 50 | Nauru |
| 51 | 45 | 53 | 44 | 44 | 37 | 44 | 28 | 29 | 17 | 26 | 20 | 20 | 19 | 18 | New Caledonia |
| 10 | 11 | 9 | 9 | 10 | 12 | 9 | 10 | 8 | 10 | 9 | 8 | 8 | 7 | 7 | New Zealand |
| 88 | 0 | 91 | 0 | 0 | 51 | 0 | 0 | 228 | 0 | 0 | 0 | 0 | 0 | 0 | Niue |
| 83 | 83 | 85 | 149 | 150 | 99 | 109 | 81 | 72 | 59 | 68 | 71 | 62 | 52 | 33 | Commonwealth of the Northern Mariana Islands |
| 247 | 111 | 29 | 83 | | 169 | | | 56 | 45 | 25 | 50 | 59 | 54 | 0 | Palau |
| 116 | 171 | 66 | 161 | 221 | 248 | 195 | 229 | 198 | 221 | 215 | 207 | 203 | 237 | 213 | Papua New Guinea |
| 268 | 174 | 236 | 273 | 222 | 195 | 157 | 138 | 149 | 164 | 158 | 162 | 171 | 160 | 155 | Philippines |
| 86 | 94 | 87 | 73 | 75 | 69 | 47 | 79 | 74 | 71 | 72 | 80 | 79 | 78 | 77 | Republic of Korea |
| 27 | 27 | 18 | 19 | 13 | 18 | 24 | 12 | 17 | 15 | 19 | 13 | 13 | | 7 | Samoa |
| 50 | 54 | 54 | 53 | 56 | 46 | 43 | 37 | 36 | 37 | 33 | 31 | 30 | 31 | 34 | Singapore |
| 94 | 97 | 80 | 83 | 75 | 71 | 73 | 68 | 58 | 65 | 74 | 84 | 77 | 80 | 76 | Solomon Islands |
| 0 | 135 | 0 | | | 0 | 0 | 0 | | 0 | | 0 | 0 | 0 | 0 | Tokelau |
| 24 | 21 | 23 | 21 | 31 | 22 | 24 | 12 | 29 | 16 | 12 | 18 | 18 | 23 | 13 | Tonga |
| 195 | 367 | | | 179 | 138 | 157 | 156 | 126 | 290 | | 115 | 86 | 171 | 170 | Tuvalu |
| 90 | 46 | 72 | 103 | 98 | 65 | 80 | 90 | 51 | 51 | 55 | 35 | 57 | 54 | 44 | Vanuatu |
| 72 | 76 | 100 | 103 | 114 | 114 | 114 | 113 | 117 | 112 | 117 | 112 | 113 | 111 | 112 | Viet Nam |
| 77 | 42 | 55 | 96 | | | | 7 | 127 | 100 | | 46 | | 13 | 0 | Wallis and Futuna |
| **46** | **51** | **54** | **53** | **50** | **49** | **47** | **47** | **47** | **57** | **67** | **73** | **75** | **77** | **76** | **Western Pacific Region** |

**Table 56.** New smear-positive cases notified, numbers and rates, 1993–2008

| | Number of cases | | | | | | | | | | | | | | | |
|---|---|---|---|---|---|---|---|---|---|---|---|---|---|---|---|---|
| | 1993 | 1994 | 1995 | 1996 | 1997 | 1998 | 1999 | 2000 | 2001 | 2002 | 2003 | 2004 | 2005 | 2006 | 2007 | 2008 |
| American Samoa | 1 | 4 | | | 6 | 2 | 3 | 2 | 2 | 1 | 2 | 2 | 3 | 3 | | |
| Australia | 557 | | | | 226 | 203 | 285 | 251 | 228 | 210 | 113 | 285 | 241 | 269 | 281 | 299 |
| Brunei Darussalam | 68 | | | | | | 102 | 84 | 95 | 112 | 121 | 115 | 101 | 128 | 136 | 132 |
| Cambodia | | 11 058 | 11 101 | 12 065 | 12 686 | 13 865 | 15 744 | 14 822 | 14 361 | 17 258 | 18 923 | 18 978 | 21 001 | 19 294 | 19 421 | 19 860 |
| China | 84 898 | 104 729 | 134 488 | 203 670 | 236 021 | 202 817 | 201 775 | 204 765 | 204 591 | 194 972 | 267 414 | 384 886 | 472 719 | 468 291 | 465 877 | 462 596 |
| Cook Islands | 5 | 4 | 2 | 1 | 2 | | | | 2 | 1 | | 1 | 1 | | 1501 | 2 |
| Fiji | 61 | 62 | 68 | 69 | 66 | 74 | 65 | 62 | 73 | 74 | 78 | 62 | 63 | 73 | 138 | 78 |
| French Polynesia | | 38 | | 37 | 41 | 34 | 33 | 29 | | 28 | 21 | 30 | 21 | 24 | | 20 |
| Guam | | 40 | | | | | | 43 | 47 | 31 | | 22 | 27 | 21 | 52 | 31 |
| Hong Kong (China) | 2429 | | | 1774 | 1943 | 2091 | 1536 | 1940 | 1857 | 1892 | 1794 | 1693 | 1561 | 1547 | 19 | 1 459 |
| Japan | 17 890 | 16 770 | 14 367 | 12 867 | 13 571 | 11 935 | 12 909 | 11 853 | 11 408 | 10 807 | 10 843 | 10 471 | 10 931 | 10 159 | 5 | 8 995 |
| Kiribati | 99 | 184 | | 144 | 50 | 52 | 59 | 54 | 64 | 82 | 99 | 142 | 124 | 129 | 9 433 | 147 |
| Lao People's Democratic Republic | | | 478 | 886 | 1234 | 1494 | 1706 | 1526 | 1563 | 1829 | 1866 | 2226 | 2806 | 3041 | 103 | 3 079 |
| Macao (China) | 108 | | 141 | 258 | 325 | 276 | | 160 | 157 | 147 | 138 | 128 | 136 | 144 | 3 080 | 139 |
| Malaysia | 6954 | 6861 | 6688 | 7271 | 7496 | 7802 | 8207 | 8156 | 8309 | 7958 | 7989 | 7843 | 8446 | 9414 | 9 578 | 10 441 |
| Marshall Islands | 12 | | | 12 | | 11 | 17 | 11 | 15 | 18 | 20 | 39 | 48 | 45 | 19 | 28 |
| The Federated States of Micronesia | | | 9 | 14 | 9 | 14 | | 15 | 8 | 22 | 26 | 35 | 32 | 41 | 47 | 38 |
| Mongolia | | 145 | 455 | 769 | 1171 | 1356 | 1513 | 1389 | 1631 | 1670 | 1541 | 1808 | 1868 | 2129 | 1 856 | 1 838 |
| Nauru | | 2 | | | | | 2 | 4 | 2 | 2 | 1 | | | 2 | 3 | 2 |
| New Caledonia | 16 | 28 | 21 | 26 | 24 | 26 | 22 | 20 | 19 | 21 | 12 | 15 | 16 | 9 | 12 | 9 |
| New Zealand | 91 | 61 | 78 | 90 | 83 | 106 | 94 | 74 | 68 | 88 | 106 | 111 | 83 | 97 | 81 | 101 |
| Niue | | | | 1 | | | 1 | | | 1 | | | | | | |
| Commonwealth of the Northern Mariana Islands | | | 14 | 26 | 21 | 26 | 15 | 27 | 19 | 21 | 16 | 14 | 15 | 15 | 14 | 13 |
| Palau | 8 | 11 | 9 | 4 | 7 | | 20 | | | 9 | 5 | 5 | 3 | 6 | 5 | |
| Papua New Guinea | | | 1652 | 447 | 1195 | 2107 | 2140 | 1933 | 1351 | 1345 | 2310 | 1896 | 1805 | 1948 | 2 087 | 2 323 |
| Philippines | 92 279 | 87 401 | 94 768 | 86 695 | 80 163 | 69 476 | 73 373 | 67 056 | 59 341 | 65 148 | 72 670 | 78 163 | 81 647 | 85 740 | 86 566 | 85 025 |
| Republic of Korea | 16 630 | 13 266 | 11 754 | 11 420 | 9957 | 10 359 | 9559 | 8216 | 11 805 | 11 345 | 10 976 | 11 471 | 11 638 | 11 513 | 10 927 | 11 048 |
| Samoa | 21 | 18 | 15 | 9 | 14 | 7 | 17 | 13 | 11 | 19 | 12 | 11 | 11 | 13 | | 6 |
| Singapore | 513 | 861 | 455 | 519 | 436 | 482 | 465 | 248 | 357 | 549 | 583 | 501 | 552 | 538 | 504 | 526 |
| Solomon Islands | 155 | 114 | 109 | 90 | 113 | 140 | 93 | 109 | 118 | 108 | 138 | 152 | 169 | 124 | 142 | 140 |
| Tokelau | | | 1 | | | | | | | | | | | | | |
| Tonga | 16 | 17 | 9 | 14 | 11 | 16 | 10 | 15 | 8 | 23 | 11 | 8 | 11 | 14 | 14 | 11 |
| Tuvalu | 2 | 1 | 6 | | | | | | | | | | 5 | 4 | 12 | 9 |
| Vanuatu | | 62 | 30 | 50 | 66 | 38 | 43 | 63 | 57 | 38 | 40 | 59 | 35 | 42 | 41 | 45 |
| Viet Nam | | | 37 550 | 48 911 | 50 016 | 54 889 | 53 805 | 53 169 | 54 238 | 56 698 | 55 937 | 58 394 | 55 492 | 56 437 | 54 457 | 53 484 |
| Wallis and Futuna | | | 3 | 3 | 1 | | | | 1 | 1 | 7 | | 1 | | 1 | |
| **Western Pacific Republic** | **222 813** | **241 737** | **314 271** | **388 142** | **416 954** | **379 698** | **383 613** | **376 109** | **371 806** | **372 528** | **453 812** | **579 566** | **671 612** | **671 254** | **666 412** | **661 924** |

Rates are per 100 000 population. The table includes updated information; data shown here may differ from those published in previous reports. Data can be downloaded from http://stoptb.wpro.who.int/.

| Rate (per 100 000 population) | | | | | | | | | | | | | | | | |
|---|---|---|---|---|---|---|---|---|---|---|---|---|---|---|---|---|
| 1993 | 1994 | 1995 | 1996 | 1997 | 1998 | 1999 | 2000 | 2001 | 2002 | 2003 | 2004 | 2005 | 2006 | 2007 | 2008 | |
| 2 | 8 | | 0 | 11 | 4 | 5 | 4 | 3 | 2 | 3 | 3 | 5 | 5 | 0 | 0 | American Samoa |
| 3 | | | | 1 | 1 | 2 | 1 | 1 | 1 | 1 | 1 | 1 | 1 | 1 | 1 | Australia |
| 24 | | | | 0 | | 31 | 25 | 28 | 32 | 34 | 31 | 27 | 34 | 35 | 34 | Brunei Darussalam |
| | 100 | 97 | 103 | 106 | 113 | 126 | 116 | 110 | 130 | 140 | 138 | 150 | 136 | 134 | 136 | Cambodia |
| 7 | 9 | 11 | 17 | 19 | 16 | 16 | 16 | 16 | 15 | 21 | 29 | 36 | 35 | 35 | 35 | China |
| 28 | 22 | 11 | 6 | 11 | 0 | 0 | 0 | 13 | 7 | 0 | 7 | 7 | 0 | | 10 | Cook Islands |
| 8 | 8 | 9 | 9 | 8 | 9 | 8 | 8 | 9 | 9 | 10 | 8 | 8 | 9 | 6 | 9 | Fiji |
| | 18 | | 17 | 18 | 15 | 14 | 12 | 0 | 11 | 8 | 12 | 8 | 9 | 7 | 8 | French Polynesia |
| | 28 | | | | | | 28 | 30 | 19 | 0 | 13 | 16 | 12 | 3 | 18 | Guam |
| 41 | | 0 | 28 | 30 | 32 | 23 | 29 | 28 | 28 | 26 | 24 | 22 | 22 | 21 | 21 | Hong Kong (China) |
| 14 | 13 | 11 | 10 | 11 | 9 | 10 | 9 | 9 | 8 | 8 | 8 | 9 | 8 | 7 | 7 | Japan |
| 132 | 241 | | 184 | 63 | 64 | 71 | 64 | 75 | 94 | 112 | 157 | 135 | 138 | 108 | 133 | Kiribati |
| | | 10 | 18 | 25 | 30 | 33 | 29 | 29 | 34 | 34 | 40 | 50 | 53 | 53 | 53 | The Lao People's Democratic Republic |
| 27 | | 34 | 62 | 77 | 64 | | 36 | 35 | 32 | 30 | 27 | 29 | 30 | 29 | 29 | Macao (China) |
| 36 | 34 | 32 | 34 | 35 | 35 | 36 | 35 | 35 | 33 | 32 | 31 | 33 | 36 | 36 | 39 | Malaysia |
| 24 | | | 23 | | 21 | 33 | 21 | 28 | 34 | 37 | 70 | 85 | 78 | 32 | 46 | Marshall Islands |
| | | 8 | 13 | 8 | 13 | | 14 | 7 | 20 | 24 | 32 | 29 | 37 | 42 | 39 | The Federated States of Micronesia |
| 0 | 6 | 19 | 32 | 48 | 56 | 62 | 56 | 66 | 67 | 61 | 71 | 72 | 82 | 71 | 70 | Mongolia |
| | 20 | | | | | 20 | 40 | 20 | 20 | 10 | | 0 | 20 | 30 | 20 | Nauru |
| 9 | 15 | 11 | 13 | 12 | 13 | 10 | 9 | 9 | 9 | 5 | 7 | 7 | 4 | 5 | 4 | New Caledonia |
| 3 | 2 | 2 | 2 | 2 | 3 | 2 | 2 | 2 | 2 | 3 | 3 | 2 | 2 | 2 | 2 | New Zealand |
| 0 | 0 | 0 | 45 | 0 | 0 | 51 | 0 | 0 | 57 | 0 | 0 | 0 | 0 | 0 | 0 | Niue |
| | | 24 | 43 | 34 | 40 | 22 | 39 | 27 | 29 | 21 | 18 | 19 | 18 | 17 | 15 | Commonwealth of the Northern Mariana Islands |
| 50 | 66 | 53 | 23 | 39 | | 106 | | | 46 | 25 | 25 | 15 | 30 | 25 | 0 | Palau |
| | | 35 | 9 | 24 | 41 | 41 | 36 | 24 | 24 | 40 | 32 | 30 | 31 | 33 | 35 | Papua New Guinea |
| 141 | 130 | 138 | 124 | 112 | 95 | 98 | 88 | 76 | 82 | 90 | 94 | 97 | 99 | 98 | 94 | Philippines |
| 38 | 30 | 26 | 25 | 22 | 22 | 21 | 18 | 25 | 24 | 23 | 24 | 24 | 24 | 23 | 23 | Republic of Korea |
| 13 | 11 | 9 | 5 | 8 | 4 | 10 | 7 | 6 | 11 | 7 | 6 | 6 | 7 | | 3 | Samoa |
| 16 | 26 | 13 | 14 | 12 | 13 | 12 | 6 | 9 | 13 | 14 | 12 | 13 | 12 | 11 | 11 | Singapore |
| 45 | 32 | 30 | 24 | 30 | 36 | 23 | 26 | 28 | 25 | 31 | 33 | 36 | 26 | 29 | 27 | Solomon Islands |
| | 0 | 68 | 0 | | | 0 | 0 | 0 | | 0 | | 0 | 0 | 0 | 0 | Tokelau |
| 17 | 18 | 9 | 14 | 11 | 16 | 10 | 15 | 8 | 23 | 11 | 8 | 11 | 14 | 14 | 11 | Tonga |
| 21 | 10 | 61 | | | | 0 | 0 | 0 | 0 | 0 | | 48 | 38 | 114 | 90 | Tuvalu |
| | 37 | 17 | 28 | 37 | 21 | 23 | 33 | 29 | 19 | 20 | 28 | 16 | 19 | 18 | 19 | Vanuatu |
| | | 51 | 66 | 66 | 71 | 69 | 67 | 68 | 70 | 68 | 70 | 65 | 65 | 62 | 61 | Viet Nam |
| | | 21 | 21 | 7 | | | | 7 | 7 | 47 | | 7 | | 7 | 0 | Wallis and Futuna |
| **14** | **15** | **20** | **24** | **25** | **23** | **23** | **22** | **22** | **22** | **26** | **33** | **38** | **38** | **38** | **37** | **Western Pacific Republic** |

# **Annex 8:** Sub-national notification data (all forms of TB) for seven countries with a high-burden of TB

| | Sub-national area | All forms of TB notified | |
|---|---|---|---|
| | | Number | Rate per 100 000 population |
| **Cambodia** | Banteay Meanchey | 1 782 | 270 |
| | Battambang | 2 011 | 204 |
| | Kampong Cham | 4 455 | 260 |
| | Kampong Chhnang | 1 180 | 246 |
| | Kampong Speu | 1 927 | 260 |
| | Kampong Thom | 1 721 | 265 |
| | Kampot | 1 632 | 276 |
| | Kandal | 3 465 | 270 |
| | Kep | 60 | 169 |
| | Koh Kong | 198 | 170 |
| | Kratie | 602 | 210 |
| | Mondul Kiri | 34 | 56 |
| | Oddar Meanchey | 399 | 215 |
| | Pailin | 241 | 403 |
| | Phnom Penh | 2 851 | 215 |
| | Preah Vihear | 323 | 189 |
| | Prey Veng | 4 846 | 438 |
| | Pursat | 1 298 | 328 |
| | Ratanak Kiri | 99 | 65 |
| | Siemreap | 3 485 | 384 |
| | Kampong Som | 444 | 244 |
| | Stung Treng | 197 | 173 |
| | Svay Rieng | 2 576 | 460 |
| | Takeo | 3 101 | 338 |
| | | | |
| **China** | Beijing | 2 526 | 15 |
| | Tianjin | 4 512 | 40 |
| | Hebei | 40 555 | 58 |
| | Shanxi | 23 864 | 70 |
| | Inner Mongolia | 23 425 | 97 |
| | Liaoning | 25 700 | 60 |
| | Jilin | 21 910 | 80 |
| | Heilongjiang | 39 045 | 102 |
| | Shanghai | 7 644 | 41 |
| | Jiangsu | 45 816 | 60 |
| | Zhejiang | 36 674 | 72 |
| | Anhui | 43 125 | 70 |
| | Fujian | 23 878 | 67 |
| | Jiangxi | 35 311 | 81 |
| | Shandong | 42 468 | 45 |
| | Henan | 82 520 | 88 |
| | Hubei | 48 073 | 84 |

| | Sub-national area | All forms of TB notified | |
|---|---|---|---|
| | | Number | Rate per 100 000 population |
| | Hunan | 51 224 | 81 |
| | Guangdong | 69 658 | 74 |
| | Guangxi | 44 497 | 93 |
| | Hainan | 9 031 | 107 |
| | Chongqing | 26 027 | 92 |
| | Sichuan | 68 507 | 84 |
| | Guizhou | 46 286 | 123 |
| | Yunnan | 20 668 | 46 |
| | Xizang | 4 555 | 160 |
| | Shaanxi | 24 143 | 64 |
| | Gansu | 24 421 | 93 |
| | Qinghai | 4 986 | 90 |
| | Ningxia | 3 526 | 58 |
| | Xinjiang | 28 383 | 121 |
| | | | |
| **Lao People's Democratic Republic** | Vientiane Municipality | 797 | 108 |
| | Phongsaly | 35 | 20 |
| | Luangnamtha | 115 | 75 |
| | Oudomxay | 175 | 81 |
| | Bokeo | 132 | 82 |
| | Luangprabang | 170 | 39 |
| | Huaphanh | 35 | 12 |
| | Xayabury | 143 | 39 |
| | Xiengkhuang | 27 | 11 |
| | Vientiane | 227 | 52 |
| | Borikhamxay | 88 | 37 |
| | Khammuane | 327 | 91 |
| | Savannakhet | 931 | 101 |
| | Saravane | 237 | 68 |
| | Sekong | 52 | 52 |
| | Champasack | 522 | 77 |
| | Attapeu | 108 | 91 |
| | | | |
| **Mongolia** | Arhangay | 79 | 85 |
| | Bayan-Olgiy | 76 | 75 |
| | Bayanhongor | 24 | 28 |
| | Bulgan | 55 | 90 |
| | Dornod | 217 | 296 |
| | Dornogovi | 70 | 124 |
| | Dundgovi | 26 | 54 |
| | Zavkhan | 24 | 30 |
| | Govi-Altay | 28 | 47 |
| | Hentiy | 168 | 236 |
| | Hovd | 48 | 54 |
| | Hovsgol | 123 | 100 |

| | Sub-national area | All forms of TB notified | |
|---|---|---|---|
| | | Number | Rate per 100 000 population |
| | Omnogovi | 27 | 57 |
| | Ovorhangay | 63 | 54 |
| | Selenge | 302 | 299 |
| | Suhbaatar | 117 | 213 |
| | Tov | 101 | 117 |
| | Uvs | 45 | 56 |
| | Govisumber | 24 | 189 |
| | Orkhon | 108 | 133 |
| | Darkhan-Uul | 261 | 297 |
| | Ulaanbaatar | 2 504 | 239 |
| | | | |
| **Papua New Guinea** | National Capital District | 3 816 | 1131 |
| | Central | 705 | 319 |
| | Eastern Highlands | 1 034 | 121 |
| | East New Britain | 814 | 311 |
| | East Sepik | 537 | 131 |
| | Enga | 232 | 63 |
| | Gulf | 747 | 569 |
| | Madang | 586 | 130 |
| | Manus | 18 | 34 |
| | Milne Bay | 607 | 237 |
| | Morobe | 1 533 | 228 |
| | North Solomons | 467 | 237 |
| | New Ireland | 179 | 120 |
| | Oro | 346 | 210 |
| | Southern Highlands | 266 | 35 |
| | Simbu | 396 | 131 |
| | Western Highlands | 417 | 112 |
| | West New Britain | 1 310 | 535 |
| | West Sepik | 395 | 176 |
| | Western | 825 | 415 |
| | | | |
| **Philippines** | Autonomous region in Muslim Mindanao (ARMM) | 4 106 | 121 |
| | Cordillera Administrative region (CAR) | 1 203 | 74 |
| | National Capital region (NCR) | 19 440 | 173 |
| | Region I (Ilocos region) | 6 787 | 136 |
| | Region II (Cagayan Valley) | 4 324 | 133 |
| | Region III (Central Luzon) | 12 089 | 124 |
| | Region IV-A (Calabarzon) | 9 667 | 85 |
| | Region IV-B (Mimaropa) | 4 902 | 171 |
| | Region IX (Western Mindanao) | 5 846 | 213 |
| | Region V (Bicol region) | 11 685 | 250 |
| | Region VI (Western Visayas) | 18 241 | 250 |
| | Region VII (Central Visayas) | 11 792 | 175 |
| | Region VIII (Eastern Visayas) | 5 063 | 151 |

| | Sub-national area | All forms of TB notified | |
|---|---|---|---|
| | | Number | Rate per 100 000 population |
| | Region X (Northern Mindanao) | 6 350 | 152 |
| | Region XI (Davao Region) | 7 260 | 172 |
| | Region XII (Soccsksargen) | 6 200 | 154 |
| | Region XIII (Caraga) | 4 548 | 189 |
| | | | |
| **Viet Nam** | Ha Noi city | 2 481 | 76 |
| | Hai Phong city | 2 197 | 122 |
| | Ha Tay | 1 939 | 76 |
| | Hai Duong | 1 455 | 84 |
| | Hung Yen | 1 134 | 102 |
| | Ha Nam | 884 | 106 |
| | Nam Dinh | 1 703 | 87 |
| | Thai Binh | 1 803 | 96 |
| | Ninh Binh | 623 | 67 |
| | Ha Giang | 314 | 46 |
| | Cao Bang | 271 | 55 |
| | Lao Cai | 236 | 40 |
| | Bac Kan | 98 | 33 |
| | Lang Son | 772 | 101 |
| | Tuyen Quang | 340 | 47 |
| | Yen Bai | 307 | 41 |
| | Thai Nguyen | 797 | 70 |
| | Vinh Phuc | 471 | 47 |
| | Phu Tho | 903 | 67 |
| | Bac Giang | 2 314 | 144 |
| | Bac Ninh | 791 | 79 |
| | Quang Ninh | 1 054 | 95 |
| | Lai Chau | 132 | 37 |
| | Dien Bien | 152 | 28 |
| | Son La | 341 | 33 |
| | Hoa Binh | 480 | 58 |
| | Thanh Hoa | 3 758 | 104 |
| | Nghe An | 2 515 | 79 |
| | Ha Tinh | 1 440 | 110 |
| | Quang Binh | 948 | 111 |
| | Quang Tri | 536 | 84 |
| | Thua Thien - Hue | 1 255 | 102 |
| | Da Nang City | 1 443 | 177 |
| | Quang Nam | 1 527 | 102 |
| | Quang Ngai | 1 242 | 93 |
| | Binh Dinh | 2 010 | 131 |
| | Phu Yen | 810 | 95 |
| | Khanh Hoa | 1 268 | 107 |
| | Kon Tum | 319 | 78 |
| | Gia Lai | 564 | 48 |

| | Sub-national area | All forms of TB notified | |
|---|---|---|---|
| | | Number | Rate per 100 000 population |
| | Dac Nong | 209 | 48 |
| | Dak Lak | 866 | 50 |
| | Ho Chi Minh city | 13 506 | 203 |
| | Lam Dong | 526 | 45 |
| | Ninh Thuan | 775 | 135 |
| | Binh Phuoc | 847 | 108 |
| | Tay Ninh | 2 119 | 201 |
| | Binh Duong | 1 742 | 154 |
| | Dong Nai | 3 126 | 138 |
| | Binh Thuan | 1 515 | 130 |
| | Ba Ria - Vung Tau | 1 357 | 136 |
| | Long An | 1 977 | 136 |
| | Dong Thap | 2 789 | 164 |
| | An Giang | 4 517 | 202 |
| | Tien Giang | 1 999 | 117 |
| | Vinh Long | 1 330 | 123 |
| | Ben Tre | 1 338 | 97 |
| | Kien Giang | 2 536 | 145 |
| | Can Tho | 1 924 | 166 |
| | Tra Vinh | 1 399 | 132 |
| | Soc Trang | 1 837 | 139 |
| | Bac Lieu | 994 | 117 |
| | Ca Mau | 1 318 | 104 |
| | Hau Giang | 1 105 | 137 |

# Annex 9: Notified prevalence of resistance to anti-TB drugs (2000–2008)

**Table 57.** Notified prevalence of resistance to specific drugs among new TB cases tested for resistance

| Country and Area | Sub-national | Year | Method | Patients tested | Suscep-tible | % | Any resis-tance | % | Any H | % | Any R | % | Any E | % | Any S | % | Mono | % | Mono H | % | Mono R | % |
|---|---|---|---|---|---|---|---|---|---|---|---|---|---|---|---|---|---|---|---|---|---|---|
| Australia | Countrywide | 2008 | Surveillance | combined only | | . | | . | | . | | . | | . | | . | | . | | . | | . |
| Cambodia | Countrywide | 2001 | Survey | 638 | 572 | 89.7 | 66 | 10.3 | 41 | 6.4 | 4 | 0.6 | 1 | 0.2 | 32 | 5.0 | 54 | 8.5 | 30 | 4.7 | 3 | 0.5 |
| China | Beijing | 2004 | Survey | 1043 | 856 | 82.1 | 187 | 17.9 | 91 | 8.7 | 44 | 4.2 | 43 | 4.1 | 95 | 9.1 | 113 | 10.8 | 35 | 3.4 | 11 | 1.1 |
| China | Henan | 2001 | Survey | 1222 | 858 | 70.2 | 364 | 29.8 | 208 | 17.0 | 117 | 9.6 | 53 | 4.3 | 271 | 22.2 | 190 | 15.5 | 40 | 3.3 | 17 | 1.4 |
| China | Heilongjiang | 2004 | Survey | 1574 | 1005 | 63.9 | 569 | 36.1 | 266 | 16.9 | 167 | 10.6 | 93 | 5.9 | 383 | 24.3 | 340 | 21.6 | 61 | 3.9 | 34 | 2.2 |
| China | Shanghai | 2004 | Survey | 764 | 646 | 84.6 | 118 | 15.4 | 89 | 11.6 | 37 | 4.8 | 23 | 3.0 | 62 | 8.1 | 57 | 7.5 | 25 | 3.3 | 6 | 0.8 |
| China | Inner Mongolia | 2002 | Survey | 876 | 592 | 67.6 | 284 | 32.4 | 164 | 18.7 | 84 | 9.6 | 72 | 8.2 | 187 | 21.3 | 148 | 16.9 | 40 | 4.6 | 13 | 1.5 |
| Fiji | Countrywide | 2006 | Surveillance | combined only | | . | | . | | . | | . | | . | | . | | . | | . | | . |
| Guam | Countrywide | 2002 | Survey | combined only | | . | | . | | . | | . | | . | | . | | . | | . | | . |
| Hong Kong (China) | Hong Kong | 2008 | Surveillance | 2443 | 2213 | 90.6 | 230 | 9.4 | 104 | 4.3 | 17 | 0.7 | 12 | 0.5 | 167 | 6.8 | 175 | 7.2 | 51 | 2.1 | 7 | 0.3 |
| Japan | Countrywide | 2007 | Surveillance | combined only | | . | | . | | . | | . | | . | | . | | . | | . | | . |
| Macao (China) | Macao | 2008 | Surveillance | 243 | 222 | 91.4 | 21 | 8.6 | 6 | 2.5 | 6 | 2.5 | 4 | 1.6 | 15 | 6.2 | 13 | 5.3 | 5 | 2.1 | 1 | 0.4 |
| New Caledonia | Countrywide | 2005 | Survey | combined only | | . | | . | | . | | . | | . | | . | | . | | . | | . |
| New Zealand | Countrywide | 2006 | Surveillance | 250 | 224 | 89.6 | 26 | 10.4 | 17 | 6.8 | 1 | 0.4 | 1 | 0.4 | 18 | 7.2 | 17 | 6.8 | 8 | 3.2 | 0 | 0.0 |
| Common-wealth of the Northern Mariana Islands | Countrywide | 2006 | Surveillance | 18 | 4 | 22.2 | 4 | 22.2 | 3 | 16.7 | 2 | 11.1 | 0 | 0.0 | 2 | 11.1 | 1 | 5.6 | 0 | 0.0 | 0 | 0.0 |
| Philippines | Countrywide | 2004 | Survey | 965 | 767 | 79.5 | 198 | 20.5 | 130 | 13.5 | 44 | 4.6 | 41 | 4.2 | 115 | 11.9 | 122 | 12.6 | 57 | 5.9 | 4 | 0.4 |
| Republic of Korea | Countrywide | 2008 | Survey | 2581 | 2276 | 88.2 | 305 | 11.8 | 248 | 9.6 | 94 | 3.6 | 66 | 2.6 | 94 | 3.6 | 184 | 7.1 | 129 | 5.0 | 13 | 0.5 |
| Singapore | Countrywide | 2008 | Surveillance | 919 | 861 | 93.7 | 58 | 6.3 | 21 | 2.3 | 1 | 0.1 | 3 | 0.3 | 46 | 5.0 | 47 | 5.1 | 10 | 1.1 | 0 | 0.0 |
| Solomon Islands | Countrywide | 2004 | Survey | combined only | | . | | . | | . | | . | | . | | . | | . | | . | | . |
| Vanuatu | Countrywide | 2006 | Surveillance | 29 | 28 | 96.6 | 1 | 3.4 | 1 | 3.4 | 0 | 0.0 | 0 | 0.0 | 0 | 0.0 | 1 | 3.4 | 1 | 3.4 | 0 | 0.0 |
| Viet Nam | Countrywide | 2006 | Survey | 1619 | 1122 | 69.3 | 497 | 30.7 | 310 | 19.1 | 53 | 3.3 | 42 | 2.6 | 375 | 23.2 | 291 | 18.0 | 114 | 7.0 | 5 | 0.3 |

H = isoniazid; R = rifampicin; E = ethanbutol; S = streptomicin; Mono = mono-resistant to; HR = resistant only to H and R; HRE = resistant to H, R and E; HRS = resistant to H, R and S; HRES = resistant to H, R, E, and S; Poly =resistant to more than one drug other than MDR; HE = resistant to H and E; HS = resistant to H and S; HES = resistant to H, E, and S; RE = resistant to R and E; RS = resistant to R and S; RES = resistant to R, E, and S; ES = resistant to E and S.

| Mono E | % | Mono S | % | MDR | % | HR | % | HRE | % | HRS | % | HRES | % | Poly | % | HE | % | HS | % | HES | % | RE | % | RS | % | RES | % | ES | % | |
|---|---|---|---|---|---|---|---|---|---|---|---|---|---|---|---|---|---|---|---|---|---|---|---|---|---|---|---|---|---|---|
| | . | | . | | . | | . | | . | | . | | . | | . | | . | | . | | . | | . | | . | | . | | . | Australia |
| 0 | 0.0 | 21 | 3.3 | 0 | 0.0 | 0 | 0.0 | 0 | 0.0 | 0 | 0.0 | 0 | 0.0 | 12 | 1.9 | 1 | 0.2 | 10 | 1.6 | 0 | 0.0 | 0 | 0.0 | 1 | 0.2 | 0 | 0.0 | 0 | 0.0 | Cambodia |
| 14 | 1.3 | 53 | 5.1 | 24 | 2.3 | 15 | 1.4 | 1 | 0.1 | 5 | 0.5 | 3 | 0.3 | 50 | 4.8 | 11 | 1.1 | 21 | 2.0 | 0 | 0.0 | 5 | 0.5 | 4 | 0.4 | 0 | 0.0 | 9 | 0.9 | China |
| 10 | 0.8 | 123 | 10.1 | 95 | 7.8 | 18 | 1.5 | 5 | 0.4 | 47 | 3.8 | 25 | 2.0 | 79 | 6.5 | 2 | 0.2 | 62 | 5.1 | 9 | 0.7 | 1 | 0.1 | 4 | 0.3 | 0 | 0.0 | 1 | 0.1 | China |
| 3 | 0.2 | 242 | 15.4 | 113 | 7.2 | 24 | 1.5 | 63 | 4.0 | 4 | 0.3 | 22 | 1.4 | 116 | 7.4 | 0 | 0.0 | 93 | 5.9 | 1 | 0.1 | 1 | 0.1 | 18 | 1.1 | 1 | 0.1 | 2 | 0.1 | China |
| 0 | 0.0 | 26 | 3.4 | 30 | 3.9 | 7 | 0.9 | 17 | 2.2 | 1 | 0.1 | 5 | 0.7 | 31 | 4.1 | 1 | 0.1 | 29 | 3.8 | 0 | 0.0 | 0 | 0.0 | 1 | 0.1 | 0 | 0.0 | 0 | 0.0 | China |
| 5 | 0.6 | 90 | 10.3 | 61 | 7.0 | 13 | 1.5 | 29 | 3.3 | 4 | 0.5 | 13 | 1.5 | 75 | 8.6 | 9 | 1.0 | 44 | 5.0 | 12 | 1.4 | 1 | 0.1 | 6 | 0.7 | 0 | 0.0 | 3 | 0.3 | China |
| | . | | . | | . | | . | | . | | . | | . | | . | | . | | . | | . | | . | | . | | . | | . | Fiji |
| | . | | . | | . | | . | | . | | . | | . | | . | | . | | . | | . | | . | | . | | . | | . | Guam |
| 1 | 0.0 | 116 | 4.7 | 8 | 0.3 | 1 | 0.0 | 0 | 0.0 | 3 | 0.1 | 4 | 0.2 | 47 | 1.9 | 3 | 0.1 | 40 | 1.6 | 2 | 0.1 | 0 | 0.0 | 0 | 0.0 | 2 | 0.1 | 0 | 0.0 | Hong Kong (China) |
| | . | | . | | . | | . | | . | | . | | . | | . | | . | | . | | . | | . | | . | | . | | . | Japan |
| 0 | 0.0 | 7 | 2.9 | 5 | 2.1 | 0 | 0.0 | 0 | 0.0 | 1 | 0.4 | 4 | 1.6 | 3 | 1.2 | 0 | 0.0 | 3 | 1.2 | 0 | 0.0 | 0 | 0.0 | 0 | 0.0 | 0 | 0.0 | 0 | 0.0 | Macao (China) |
| | . | | . | | . | | . | | . | | . | | . | | . | | . | | . | | . | | . | | . | | . | | . | New Caledonia |
| 0 | 0.0 | 9 | 3.6 | 1 | 0.4 | 0 | 0.0 | 0 | 0.0 | 0 | 0.0 | 1 | 0.4 | 8 | 3.2 | 0 | 0.0 | 8 | 3.2 | 0 | 0.0 | 0 | 0.0 | 0 | 0.0 | 0 | 0.0 | 0 | 0.0 | New Zealand |
| 0 | 0.0 | 1 | 5.6 | 2 | 11.1 | 2 | 11.1 | 0 | 0.0 | 0 | 0.0 | 0 | 0.0 | 1 | 5.6 | 0 | 0.0 | 1 | 5.6 | 0 | 0.0 | 0 | 0.0 | 0 | 0.0 | 0 | 0.0 | 0 | 0.0 | Commonwealth of the Northern Mariana Islands |
| 1 | 0.1 | 60 | 6.2 | 39 | 4.0 | 10 | 1.0 | 5 | 0.5 | 5 | 0.5 | 19 | 2.0 | 37 | 3.8 | 5 | 0.5 | 21 | 2.2 | 8 | 0.8 | 1 | 0.1 | 0 | 0.0 | 0 | 0.0 | 2 | 0.2 | Philippines |
| 6 | 0.2 | 36 | 1.4 | 79 | 3.1 | 29 | 1.1 | 23 | 0.9 | 7 | 0.3 | 20 | 0.8 | 42 | 1.6 | 9 | 0.3 | 25 | 1.0 | 6 | 0.2 | 2 | 0.1 | 0 | 0.0 | 0 | 0.0 | 0 | 0.0 | Republic of Korea |
| 0 | 0.0 | 37 | 4.0 | 1 | 0.1 | 0 | 0.0 | 0 | 0.0 | 0 | 0.0 | 1 | 0.1 | 10 | 1.1 | 2 | 0.2 | 8 | 0.9 | 0 | 0.0 | 0 | 0.0 | 0 | 0.0 | 0 | 0.0 | 0 | 0.0 | Singapore |
| | . | | . | | . | | . | | . | | . | | . | | . | | . | | . | | . | | . | | . | | . | | . | Solomon Islands |
| 0 | 0.0 | 0 | 0.0 | 0 | 0.0 | 0 | 0.0 | 0 | 0.0 | 0 | 0.0 | 0 | 0.0 | 0 | 0.0 | 0 | 0.0 | 0 | 0.0 | 0 | 0.0 | 0 | 0.0 | 0 | 0.0 | 0 | 0.0 | 0 | 0.0 | Vanuatu |
| 3 | 0.2 | 169 | 10.4 | 44 | 2.7 | 0 | 0.0 | 0 | 0.0 | 20 | 1.2 | 24 | 1.5 | 162 | 10.0 | 0 | 0.0 | 143 | 8.8 | 9 | 0.6 | 0 | 0.0 | 4 | 0.2 | 0 | 0.0 | 6 | 0.4 | Viet Nam |

**Table 58.** Notified prevalence of resistance to specific drugs among previously treated TB cases tested for resistance

| Country and Area | Sub-national | Year | Method | Patients tested | Suscep-tible | % | Any resis-tance | % | Any H | % | Any R | % | Any E | % | Any S | % | Mono | % | Mono H | % | Mono R | % |
|---|---|---|---|---|---|---|---|---|---|---|---|---|---|---|---|---|---|---|---|---|---|---|
| Australia | Countrywide | 2008 | Surveillance | combined only | . | | . | | . | | . | | . | | . | | . | | . | | . | |
| Cambodia | Countrywide | 2001 | Survey | 96 | 79 | 82.3 | 17 | 17.7 | 16 | 16.7 | 3 | 3.1 | 0 | 0.0 | 7 | 7.3 | 10 | 10.4 | 9 | 9.4 | 0 | 0.0 |
| China | Beijing | 2004 | Survey | 154 | 100 | 64.9 | 54 | 35.1 | 38 | 24.7 | 23 | 14.9 | 14 | 9.1 | 33 | 21.4 | 17 | 11.0 | 7 | 4.5 | 2 | 1.3 |
| China | Henan | 2001 | Survey | 265 | 104 | 39.2 | 161 | 60.8 | 125 | 47.2 | 113 | 42.6 | 48 | 18.1 | 114 | 43.0 | 38 | 14.3 | 11 | 4.2 | 8 | 3.0 |
| China | Heilongjiang | 2004 | Survey | 421 | 137 | 32.5 | 284 | 67.5 | 202 | 48.0 | 170 | 40.4 | 103 | 24.5 | 136 | 32.3 | 101 | 24.0 | 37 | 8.8 | 24 | 5.7 |
| China | Shanghai | 2004 | Survey | 200 | 145 | 72.5 | 55 | 27.5 | 43 | 21.5 | 30 | 15.0 | 20 | 10.0 | 25 | 12.5 | 19 | 9.5 | 11 | 5.5 | 2 | 1.0 |
| China | Inner Mongolia | 2002 | Survey | 386 | 157 | 40.7 | 229 | 59.3 | 218 | 56.5 | 175 | 45.3 | 123 | 31.9 | 115 | 29.8 | 52 | 13.5 | 23 | 6.0 | 16 | 4.1 |
| Fiji | Countrywide | 2006 | Surveillance | combined only | . | | . | | . | | . | | . | | . | | . | | . | | . | |
| Guam | Countrywide | 2002 | Survey | combined only | . | | . | | . | | . | | . | | . | | . | | . | | . | |
| Hong Kong (China) | Hong Kong | 2008 | Surveillance | 310 | 262 | 84.5 | 48 | 15.5 | 31 | 10.0 | 11 | 3.5 | 8 | 2.6 | 29 | 9.4 | 29 | 9.4 | 13 | 4.2 | 0 | 0.0 |
| Japan | Countrywide | 2007 | Surveillance | combined only | . | | . | | . | | . | | . | | . | | . | | . | | . | |
| Macao (China) | Macao | 2008 | Surveillance | 25 | 20 | 80.0 | 5 | 20.0 | 4 | 16.0 | 2 | 8.0 | 3 | 12.0 | 4 | 16.0 | 1 | 4.0 | 0 | 0.0 | 0 | 0.0 |
| New Caledonia | Countrywide | 2005 | Survey | combined only | . | | . | | . | | . | | . | | . | | . | | . | | . | |
| New Zealand | Countrywide | 2006 | Surveillance | 16 | 15 | 93.8 | 1 | 6.3 | 1 | 6.3 | 0 | 0.0 | 0 | 0.0 | 0 | 0.0 | 1 | 6.3 | 1 | 6.3 | 0 | 0.0 |
| Common-wealth of the Northern Mariana Islands | Countrywide | 2006 | Surveillance | new only | . | | . | | . | | . | | . | | . | | . | | . | | . | |
| Philippines | Countrywide | 2004 | Survey | 129 | 81 | 62.8 | 48 | 37.2 | 40 | 31.0 | 33 | 25.6 | 12 | 9.3 | 22 | 17.1 | 17 | 13.2 | 10 | 7.8 | 5 | 3.9 |
| Republic of Korea | Countrywide | 2008 | Survey | 731 | 564 | 77.2 | 167 | 22.8 | 145 | 19.8 | 105 | 14.4 | 51 | 7.0 | 42 | 5.7 | 63 | 8.6 | 42 | 5.7 | 14 | 1.9 |
| Singapore | Countrywide | 2008 | Surveillance | 103 | 95 | 92.2 | 8 | 7.8 | 10 | 9.7 | 3 | 2.9 | 0 | 0.0 | 9 | 8.7 | 3 | 2.9 | 5 | 4.9 | 0 | 0.0 |
| Solomon Islands | Countrywide | 2004 | Survey | combined only | . | | . | | . | | . | | . | | . | | . | | . | | . | |
| Vanuatu | Countrywide | 2006 | Surveillance | new only | . | | . | | . | | . | | . | | . | | . | | . | | . | |
| Viet Nam | Countrywide | 2006 | Survey | 207 | 85 | 41.1 | 122 | 58.9 | 90 | 43.5 | 44 | 21.3 | 30 | 14.5 | 105 | 50.7 | 38 | 18.4 | 8 | 3.9 | 2 | 1.0 |

H = isoniazid; R = rifampicin; E = ethanbutol; S = streptomicin; Mono = mono-resistant to; HR = resistant only to H and R; HRE = resistant to H, R and E;
HRS = resistant to H, R and S; HRES = resistant to H, R, E, and S; Poly = resistant to more than one drug other than MDR; HE = resistant to H and E;
HS = resistant to H and S; HES = resistant to H, E, and S; RE = resistant to R and E; RS = resistant to R and S; RES = resistant to R, E, and S;
ES = resistant to E and S.

| Mono E | % | Mono S | % | MDR | % | HR | % | HRE | % | HRS | % | HRES | % | Poly | % | HE | % | HS | % | HES | % | RE | % | RS | % | RES | % | ES | % | |
|---|---|---|---|---|---|---|---|---|---|---|---|---|---|---|---|---|---|---|---|---|---|---|---|---|---|---|---|---|---|---|
| . | | . | | . | | . | | . | | . | | . | | . | | . | | . | | . | | . | | . | | . | | . | | Australia |
| 0 | 0.0 | 1 | 1.0 | 3 | 3.1 | 1 | 1.0 | 0 | 0.0 | 2 | 2.1 | 0 | 0.0 | 4 | 4.2 | 0 | 0.0 | 4 | 4.2 | 0 | 0.0 | 0 | 0.0 | 0 | 0.0 | 0 | 0.0 | 0 | 0.0 | Cambodia |
| 0 | 0.0 | 8 | 5.2 | 18 | 11.7 | 6 | 3.9 | 2 | 1.3 | 7 | 4.5 | 3 | 1.9 | 19 | 12.3 | 3 | 1.9 | 8 | 5.2 | 2 | 1.3 | 1 | 0.6 | 2 | 1.3 | 0 | 0.0 | 3 | 1.9 | Beijing |
| 4 | 1.5 | 15 | 5.7 | 97 | 36.6 | 20 | 7.5 | 2 | 0.8 | 41 | 15.5 | 34 | 12.8 | 26 | 9.8 | 0 | 0.0 | 13 | 4.9 | 4 | 1.5 | 2 | 0.8 | 5 | 1.9 | 1 | 0.4 | 1 | 0.4 | Henan |
| 0 | 0.0 | 40 | 9.5 | 128 | 30.4 | 25 | 5.9 | 58 | 13.8 | 6 | 1.4 | 39 | 9.3 | 55 | 13.1 | 3 | 0.7 | 32 | 7.6 | 2 | 0.5 | 1 | 0.2 | 17 | 4.0 | 0 | 0.0 | 0 | 0.0 | Heilongjiang |
| 1 | 0.5 | 5 | 2.5 | 25 | 12.5 | 6 | 3.0 | 10 | 5.0 | 2 | 1.0 | 7 | 3.5 | 11 | 5.5 | 0 | 0.0 | 7 | 3.5 | 0 | 0.0 | 0 | 0.0 | 2 | 1.0 | 1 | 0.5 | 1 | 0.5 | Shanghai |
| 0 | 0.0 | 13 | 3.4 | 142 | 36.8 | 34 | 8.8 | 48 | 12.4 | 6 | 1.6 | 41 | 10.6 | 35 | 9.1 | 2 | 0.5 | 17 | 4.4 | 3 | 0.8 | 1 | 0.3 | 9 | 2.3 | 2 | 0.5 | 1 | 0.3 | Inner Mongolia |
| . | | . | | . | | . | | . | | . | | . | | . | | . | | . | | . | | . | | . | | . | | . | | Fiji |
| . | | . | | . | | . | | . | | . | | . | | . | | . | | . | | . | | . | | . | | . | | . | | Guam |
| 0 | 0.0 | 16 | 5.2 | 10 | 3.2 | 2 | 0.6 | 3 | 1.0 | 1 | 0.3 | 4 | 1.3 | 9 | 2.9 | 0 | 0.0 | 8 | 2.6 | 0 | 0.0 | 1 | 0.3 | 0 | 0.0 | 0 | 0.0 | 0 | 0.0 | Hong Kong, China |
| . | | . | | . | | . | | . | | . | | . | | . | | . | | . | | . | | . | | . | | . | | . | | Japan |
| 1 | 4.0 | 0 | 0.0 | 2 | 8.0 | 0 | 0.0 | 0 | 0.0 | 1 | 4.0 | 1 | 4.0 | 2 | 8.0 | 0 | 0.0 | 1 | 4.0 | 1 | 4.0 | 0 | 0.0 | 0 | 0.0 | 0 | 0.0 | 0 | 0.0 | Macao, China |
| . | | . | | . | | . | | . | | . | | . | | . | | . | | . | | . | | . | | . | | . | | . | | New Caledonia |
| 0 | 0.0 | 0 | 0.0 | 0 | 0.0 | 0 | 0.0 | 0 | 0.0 | 0 | 0.0 | 0 | 0.0 | 0 | 0.0 | 0 | 0.0 | 0 | 0.0 | 0 | 0.0 | 0 | 0.0 | 0 | 0.0 | 0 | 0.0 | 0 | 0.0 | New Zealand |
| . | | . | | . | | . | | . | | . | | . | | . | | . | | . | | . | | . | | . | | . | | . | | Commonwealth of the Northern Mariana Islands |
| 0 | 0.0 | 2 | 1.6 | 27 | 20.9 | 7 | 5.4 | 4 | 3.1 | 8 | 6.2 | 8 | 6.2 | 4 | 3.1 | 0 | 0.0 | 3 | 2.3 | 0 | 0.0 | 0 | 0.0 | 1 | 0.8 | 0 | 0.0 | 0 | 0.0 | Philippines |
| 1 | 0.1 | 6 | 0.8 | 90 | 12.3 | 37 | 5.1 | 25 | 3.4 | 9 | 1.2 | 19 | 2.6 | 14 | 1.9 | 5 | 0.7 | 8 | 1.1 | 0 | 0.0 | 1 | 0.1 | 0 | 0.0 | 0 | 0.0 | 0 | 0.0 | Republic of Korea |
| 0 | 0.0 | 5 | 4.9 | 3 | 2.9 | 1 | 1.0 | 0 | 0.0 | 2 | 1.9 | 0 | 0.0 | 2 | 1.9 | 0 | 0.0 | 2 | 1.9 | 0 | 0.0 | 0 | 0.0 | 0 | 0.0 | 0 | 0.0 | 0 | 0.0 | Singapore |
| . | | . | | . | | . | | . | | . | | . | | . | | . | | . | | . | | . | | . | | . | | . | | Solomon Islands |
| . | | . | | . | | . | | . | | . | | . | | . | | . | | . | | . | | . | | . | | . | | . | | Vanuatu |
| 2 | 1.0 | 26 | 12.6 | 40 | 19.3 | 5 | 2.4 | 0 | 0.0 | 15 | 7.2 | 20 | 9.7 | 44 | 21.3 | 0 | 0.0 | 34 | 16.4 | 8 | 3.9 | 0 | 0.0 | 2 | 1.0 | 0 | 0.0 | 0 | 0.0 | Viet Nam |

**Table 59.** Notified prevalence of resistance to specific drugs among all TB cases tested for resistance

| Country and Area | Sub-national | Year | Method | Patients tested | Suscep-tible | % | Any resis-tance | % | Any H | % | Any R | % | Any E | % | Any S | % | Mono | % | Mono H | % | Mono R | % |
|---|---|---|---|---|---|---|---|---|---|---|---|---|---|---|---|---|---|---|---|---|---|---|
| Australia | Countrywide | 2008 | Surveillance | 887 | 791 | 89.2 | 96 | 10.8 | 77 | 8.7 | 23 | 2.6 | 11 | 1.2 | 54 | 6.1 | 52 | 5.9 | 34 | 3.8 | 1 | 0.1 |
| Cambodia | Countrywide | 2001 | Survey | 734 | 651 | 88.7 | 83 | 11.3 | 57 | 7.8 | 7 | 1.0 | 1 | 0.1 | 39 | 5.3 | 64 | 8.7 | 39 | 5.3 | 3 | 0.4 |
| China | Beijing | 2004 | Survey | 1197 | 956 | 79.9 | 241 | 20.1 | 129 | 10.8 | 67 | 5.6 | 57 | 4.8 | 128 | 10.7 | 130 | 10.9 | 42 | 3.5 | 13 | 1.1 |
| China | Henan | 2001 | Survey | 1487 | 962 | 64.7 | 525 | 35.3 | 333 | 22.4 | 230 | 15.5 | 101 | 6.8 | 385 | 25.9 | 228 | 15.3 | 51 | 3.4 | 25 | 1.7 |
| China | Heilongjiang | 2004 | Survey | 1995 | 1142 | 57.2 | 853 | 42.8 | 468 | 23.5 | 337 | 16.9 | 196 | 9.8 | 519 | 26.0 | 441 | 22.1 | 98 | 4.9 | 58 | 2.9 |
| China | Shanghai | 2004 | Survey | 964 | 791 | 82.1 | 173 | 17.9 | 132 | 13.7 | 67 | 7.0 | 43 | 4.5 | 87 | 9.0 | 76 | 7.9 | 36 | 3.7 | 8 | 0.8 |
| China | Inner Mongolia | 2002 | Survey | 1262 | 749 | 59.4 | 513 | 40.6 | 382 | 30.3 | 259 | 20.5 | 195 | 15.5 | 302 | 23.9 | 200 | 15.8 | 63 | 5.0 | 29 | 2.3 |
| Fiji | Countrywide | 2006 | Surveillance | 38 | 38 | 100.0 | 0 | 0.0 | 0 | 0.0 | 0 | 0.0 | 0 | 0.0 | 0 | 0.0 | 0 | 0.0 | 0 | 0.0 | 0 | 0.0 |
| Guam | Countrywide | 2002 | Survey | 47 | 45 | 95.7 | 2 | 4.3 | 4 | 8.5 | 2 | 4.3 | 1 | 2.1 | 2 | 4.3 | 0 | 0.0 | 0 | 0.0 | 0 | 0.0 |
| Hong Kong (China) | Hong Kong | 2008 | Surveillance | 2753 | 2475 | 89.9 | 278 | 10.1 | 135 | 4.9 | 28 | 1.0 | 20 | 0.7 | 196 | 7.1 | 204 | 7.4 | 64 | 2.3 | 7 | 0.3 |
| Japan* | Countrywide | 2007 | Surveillance | 1859 | 1688 | 90.8 | 171 | 9.2 | 56 | 3.0 | 24 | 1.3 | 15 | 0.8 | 122 | 6.6 | 133 | 7.2 | 25 | 1.3 | 7 | 0.4 |
| Macao (China) | Macao | 2008 | Surveillance | 268 | 242 | 90.3 | 26 | 9.7 | 10 | 3.7 | 8 | 3.0 | 7 | 2.6 | 19 | 7.1 | 14 | 5.2 | 5 | 1.9 | 1 | 0.4 |
| New Caledonia | Countrywide | 2005 | Survey | 5 | 4 | 80.0 | 1 | 20.0 | 1 | 20.0 | 0 | 0.0 | 0 | 0.0 | 1 | 20.0 | 0 | 0.0 | 0 | 0.0 | 0 | 0.0 |
| New Zealand | Countrywide | 2006 | Surveillance | 266 | 239 | 89.8 | 27 | 10.2 | 18 | 6.8 | 1 | 0.4 | 1 | 0.4 | 18 | 6.8 | 18 | 6.8 | 9 | 3.4 | 0 | 0.0 |
| Commonwealth of the Northern Mariana Islands | Countrywide | 2006 | Surveillance | new only | . |  | . |  | . |  | . |  | . |  | . |  | . |  | . |  | . |  |
| Philippines | Countrywide | 2004 | Survey | 1094 | 848 | 77.5 | 246 | 22.5 | 170 | 15.5 | 77 | 7.0 | 53 | 4.8 | 137 | 12.5 | 139 | 12.7 | 67 | 6.1 | 9 | 0.8 |
| Republic of Korea | Countrywide | 2008 | Survey | 3312 | 2840 | 85.7 | 472 | 14.3 | 393 | 11.9 | 199 | 6.0 | 117 | 3.5 | 136 | 4.1 | 247 | 7.5 | 171 | 5.2 | 27 | 0.8 |
| Singapore | Countrywide | 2008 | Surveillance | 1022 | 956 | 93.5 | 66 | 6.5 | 31 | 3.0 | 4 | 0.4 | 3 | 0.3 | 55 | 5.4 | 50 | 4.9 | 15 | 1.5 | 0 | 0.0 |
| Solomon Islands | Countrywide | 2004 | Survey | 84 | 84 | 100.0 | 0 | 0.0 | 0 | 0.0 | 0 | 0.0 | 0 | 0.0 | 0 | 0.0 | 0 | 0.0 | 0 | 0.0 | 0 | 0.0 |
| Vanuatu | Countrywide | 2006 | Surveillance | new only | . |  | . |  | . |  | . |  | . |  | . |  | . |  | . |  | . |  |
| Viet Nam | Countrywide | 2006 | Survey | 1826 | 1207 | 66.1 | 619 | 33.9 | 400 | 21.9 | 97 | 5.3 | 72 | 3.9 | 480 | 26.3 | 329 | 18.0 | 122 | 6.7 | 7 | 0.4 |

H = isoniazid; R = rifampicin; E = ethanbutol; S = streptomicin; Mono = mono-resistant to; HR = resistant only to H and R; HRE = resistant to H, R and E; HRS = resistant to H, R and S; HRES = resistant to H, R, E, and S; Poly =resistant to more than one drug other than MDR; HE = resistant to H and E; HS = resistant to H and S; HES = resistant to H, E, and S; RE = resistant to R and E; RS = resistant to R and S; RES = resistant to R, E, and S; ES = resistant to E and S.

* The data from Japan is preliminary and the final data will be available in 2010.

| Mono E | % | Mono S | % | MDR | % | HR | % | HRE | % | HRS | % | HRES | % | Poly | % | HE | % | HS | % | HES | % | RE | % | RS | % | RES | % | ES | % | |
|---|---|---|---|---|---|---|---|---|---|---|---|---|---|---|---|---|---|---|---|---|---|---|---|---|---|---|---|---|---|---|
| 1 | 0.1 | 16 | 1.8 | 21 | 2.4 | 4 | 0.5 | 1 | 0.1 | 9 | 1.0 | 7 | 0.8 | 23 | 2.6 | 1 | 0.1 | 20 | 2.3 | 1 | 0.1 | 0 | 0.0 | 1 | 0.1 | 0 | 0.0 | 0 | 0.0 | Australia |
| 0 | 0.0 | 22 | 3.0 | 3 | 0.4 | 1 | 0.1 | 0 | 0.0 | 2 | 0.3 | 0 | 0.0 | 16 | 2.2 | 1 | 0.1 | 14 | 1.9 | 0 | 0.0 | 0 | 0.0 | 1 | 0.1 | 0 | 0.0 | 0 | 0.0 | Cambodia |
| 14 | 1.2 | 61 | 5.1 | 42 | 3.5 | 21 | 1.8 | 3 | 0.3 | 12 | 1.0 | 6 | 0.5 | 69 | 5.8 | 14 | 1.2 | 29 | 2.4 | 2 | 0.2 | 6 | 0.5 | 6 | 0.5 | 0 | 0.0 | 12 | 1.0 | China |
| 14 | 0.9 | 138 | 9.3 | 192 | 12.9 | 38 | 2.6 | 7 | 0.5 | 88 | 5.9 | 59 | 4.0 | 105 | 7.1 | 2 | 0.1 | 75 | 5.0 | 13 | 0.9 | 3 | 0.2 | 9 | 0.6 | 1 | 0.1 | 2 | 0.1 | China |
| 3 | 0.2 | 282 | 14.1 | 241 | 12.1 | 49 | 2.5 | 121 | 6.1 | 10 | 0.5 | 61 | 3.1 | 171 | 8.6 | 3 | 0.2 | 125 | 6.3 | 3 | 0.2 | 2 | 0.1 | 35 | 1.8 | 1 | 0.1 | 2 | 0.1 | China |
| 1 | 0.1 | 31 | 3.2 | 55 | 5.7 | 13 | 1.3 | 27 | 2.8 | 3 | 0.3 | 12 | 1.2 | 42 | 4.4 | 1 | 0.1 | 36 | 3.7 | 0 | 0.0 | 0 | 0.0 | 3 | 0.3 | 1 | 0.1 | 1 | 0.1 | China |
| 5 | 0.4 | 103 | 8.2 | 203 | 16.1 | 47 | 3.7 | 77 | 6.1 | 10 | 0.8 | 54 | 4.3 | 110 | 8.7 | 11 | 0.9 | 61 | 4.3 | 15 | 1.2 | 2 | 0.2 | 15 | 1.2 | 2 | 0.2 | 4 | 0.3 | China |
| 0 | 0.0 | 0 | 0.0 | 0 | 0.0 | 0 | 0.0 | 0 | 0.0 | 0 | 0.0 | 0 | 0.0 | 0 | 0.0 | 0 | 0.0 | 0 | 0.0 | 0 | 0.0 | 0 | 0.0 | 0 | 0.0 | 0 | 0.0 | 0 | 0.0 | Fiji |
| 0 | 0.0 | 0 | 0.0 | 2 | 4.3 | 0 | 0.0 | 0 | 0.0 | 0 | 0.0 | 0 | 0.0 | 0 | 0.0 | 0 | 0.0 | 0 | 0.0 | 0 | 0.0 | 0 | 0.0 | 0 | 0.0 | 0 | 0.0 | 0 | 0.0 | Guam |
| 1 | 0.0 | 132 | 4.8 | 18 | 0.7 | 3 | 0.1 | 3 | 0.1 | 4 | 0.1 | 8 | 0.3 | 56 | 2.0 | 3 | 0.1 | 48 | 1.7 | 2 | 0.1 | 1 | 0.0 | 0 | 0.0 | 2 | 0.1 | 0 | 0.0 | Hong Kong (China) |
| 3 | 0.2 | 98 | 5.3 | 14 | 0.8 | 5 | 0.3 | 3 | 0.2 | 3 | 0.2 | 3 | 0.2 | 24 | 1.3 | 2 | 0.1 | 16 | 0.9 | 2 | 0.1 | 1 | 0.1 | 2 | 0.1 | 0 | 0.0 | 1 | 0.1 | Japan* |
| 1 | 0.4 | 7 | 2.6 | 7 | 2.6 | 0 | 0.0 | 0 | 0.0 | 2 | 0.7 | 5 | 1.9 | 5 | 1.9 | 0 | 0.0 | 4 | 1.5 | 1 | 0.4 | 0 | 0.0 | 0 | 0.0 | 0 | 0.0 | 0 | 0.0 | Macao (China) |
| 0 | 0.0 | 0 | 0.0 | 0 | 0.0 | 0 | 0.0 | 0 | 0.0 | 0 | 0.0 | 0 | 0.0 | 1 | 20.0 | 0 | 0.0 | 1 | 20.0 | 0 | 0.0 | 0 | 0.0 | 0 | 0.0 | 0 | 0.0 | 0 | 0.0 | New Caledonia |
| 0 | 0.0 | 9 | 3.4 | 1 | 0.4 | 0 | 0.0 | 0 | 0.0 | 0 | 0.0 | 1 | 0.4 | 8 | 3.0 | 0 | 0.0 | 8 | 3.0 | 0 | 0.0 | 0 | 0.0 | 0 | 0.0 | 0 | 0.0 | 0 | 0.0 | New Zealand |
| . | | . | | . | | . | | . | | . | | . | | . | | . | | . | | . | | . | | . | | . | | . | | Commonwealth of the Northern Mariana Islands |
| 1 | 0.1 | 62 | 5.7 | 66 | 6.0 | 17 | 1.6 | 9 | 0.8 | 13 | 1.2 | 27 | 2.5 | 41 | 3.7 | 5 | 0.5 | 24 | 2.2 | 8 | 0.7 | 1 | 0.1 | 1 | 0.1 | 0 | 0.0 | 2 | 0.2 | Philippines |
| 7 | 0.2 | 42 | 1.3 | 169 | 5.1 | 66 | 2.0 | 48 | 1.4 | 16 | 0.5 | 39 | 1.2 | 56 | 1.7 | 14 | 0.4 | 33 | 1.0 | 6 | 0.2 | 3 | 0.1 | 0 | 0.0 | 0 | 0.0 | 0 | 0.0 | Republic of Korea |
| 0 | 0.0 | 42 | 4.1 | 4 | 0.4 | 1 | 0.1 | 0 | 0.0 | 2 | 0.2 | 1 | 0.1 | 12 | 1.2 | 2 | 0.2 | 10 | 1.0 | 0 | 0.0 | 0 | 0.0 | 0 | 0.0 | 0 | 0.0 | 0 | 0.0 | Singapore |
| 0 | 0.0 | 0 | 0.0 | 0 | 0.0 | 0 | 0.0 | 0 | 0.0 | 0 | 0.0 | 0 | 0.0 | 0 | 0.0 | 0 | 0.0 | 0 | 0.0 | 0 | 0.0 | 0 | 0.0 | 0 | 0.0 | 0 | 0.0 | 0 | 0.0 | Solomon Islands |
| . | | . | | . | | . | | . | | . | | . | | . | | . | | . | | . | | . | | . | | . | | . | | Vanuatu |
| 5 | 0.3 | 195 | 10.7 | 84 | 4.6 | 5 | 0.3 | 0 | 0.0 | 35 | 1.9 | 44 | 2.4 | 206 | 11.3 | 0 | 0.0 | 177 | 9.7 | 17 | 0.9 | 0 | 0.0 | 6 | 0.3 | 0 | 0.0 | 6 | 0.3 | Viet Nam |

**Table 60.** Notified prevalence of extensively drug resistance TB (XDR-TB) among MDR-TB, 2002–2008

| Country | Source | Year | Method | MDR | MDR tested | Any Resistance to FLQ | %FLQ | 95%CI | 95%CI | XDR | %XDR | 95%CI | 95%CI |
|---|---|---|---|---|---|---|---|---|---|---|---|---|---|
| Representative survey or surveillance data | | | | | | | | | | | | | |
| Japan | Global Project, SRL Japan | 2002 | sentinel | 60 | 55 | 21 | 38 | 32 | 45 | 17 | 31 | 25 | 37 |
| Hong Kong (China) | Global Project, SRL Hong Kong | 2007–2008 | surveillance | 30 | 30 | 7 | 23 | 16 | 31 | 2 | 6.7 | 2.1 | 11 |
| Republic of Korea | Global Project | 2008 | survey | 169 | 169 | 28 | 17 | 14 | 19 | 8 | 4.7 | 3.1 | 6.4 |
| Australia | Global Project, SRLs Australia | 2007–2008 | surveillance | 45 | 45 | 1 | 2 | 0 | 4.4 | 0 | 0 | | |
| Singapore | Global Project | 2006–2008 | surveillance | 14 | 14 | 0 | 0 | | | 0 | 0 | | |
| Macao (China) | Global Project | 2008 | surveillance | 7 | 7 | 1 | 14 | 1.1 | 28 | 0 | 0 | | |
| New Zealand | Global Project | 2005 | surveillance | 4 | 4 | 2 | 50 | | | 0 | 0 | | |
| | | | | | | | | | | | | | |
| Risk groups and MDR-TB treatment programmes | | | | | | | | | | | | | |
| Philippines | Global ProjectGLC program | 2005–2006 | Confirmed MDR for Tx | | 293 | 149 | 50.9 | 45 | 56.7 | 10 | 3.4 | 1.6 | 6.2 |

FLQ: fluroquinolone, CI: confidence interval, SRL: Supranational Reference Laboratory, Tx: treatment, GLC: Green Light Committee

**Table 61.** Estimated prevalence and prevalent cases of MDR-TB in selected countries and areas in the Region, 2008

| Country | Source | Year | Method | MDR | MDR tested | Any Resistance to FLQ |
|---|---|---|---|---|---|---|
| Australia | model | 2.2 (0.0–10.7) | 10.8 (0.0–34.5) | 19 (9–33) | 1 (0–2) | 21 (9–32) |
| Brunei Darussalam | model | 2.2 (0.0–10.7) | 10.8 (0.0–34.5) | 11 (0–29) | 1 (0–3) | 12 (0–26) |
| Cambodia | DRS | 0.0 (0.0–0.6) | 3.1 (1.1–8.8) | 2000 (112–4900) | 200 (0–580) | 2200 (0–4600) |
| China | DRS | 5.7 (5.0–6.6) | 25.6 (22.6–28.3) | 84 000 (65 000–106 000) | 15 000 (12 000–20 000) | 100 000 (79000–120 000) |
| Cook Islands | model | 1.9 (0.0–7.5) | 13.8 (0.0–36.2) | 0 (0–0) | 0 (0–0) | 0 (0–0) |
| Fiji | model | 1.9 (0.0–7.5) | 13.8 (0.0–36.2) | 5 (0–12) | 1 (0–2) | 5 (0–11) |
| Japan | DRS | 0.7 (0.5–1.1) | 9.8 (7.3–13.1) | 220 (130–340) | 64 (43–87) | 290 (180–390) |
| Kiribati | model | 1.9 (0.0–7.5) | 13.8 (0.0–36.2) | 10 (1–24) | 1 (0–3) | 11 (0–22) |
| Lao People's Democratic Republic | model | 1.9 (0.0–7.5) | 13.8 (0.0–36.2) | 270 (13–650) | 8 (0–23) | 280 (0–590) |
| Malaysia | DRS | 0.1 (0.0–0.6) | 0.0 (0.0–19.4) | 31 (1–120) | 74 (0–210) | 104 (0–220) |
| Marshall Islands | model | 1.9 (0.0–7.5) | 13.8 (0.0–36.2) | 4 (0–9) | 0 (0–1) | 4 (0–8) |
| Federated States of Micronesia | model | 1.9 (0.0–7.5) | 13.8 (0.0–36.2) | 3 (0–7) | 0 (0–0) | 3 (0–6) |
| Mongolia | DRS | 1.0 (0.4–2.5) | 13.8 (0.0–36.2) | 63 (17–140) | 43 (0–120) | 110 (21–190) |
| Nauru | model | 1.9 (0.0–7.5) | 13.8 (0.0–36.2) | 0 (0–0) | 0 (0–0) | 0 (0–0) |
| New Zealand | DRS | 0.0 (0.0–1.6) | 0.0 (0.0–39.0) | 15 (1–37) | 1 (0–2) | 15 (0–33) |
| Niue | model | 1.9 (0.0–7.5) | 13.8 (0.0–36.2) | - | - | - |
| Palau | model | 1.9 (0.0–7.5) | 13.8 (0.0–36.2) | 0 (0–1) | 0 (0–0) | 0 (0–1) |
| Papua New Guinea | model | 1.9 (0.0–7.5) | 13.8 (0.0–36.2) | 530 (9–1300) | 73 (0–210) | 600 (0–1200) |
| Philippines | DRS | 4.0 (3.0–5.5) | 20.9 (14.8–28.7) | 11 000 (7300–15 000) | 2000 (1100–3000) | 13 000 (8900–17 000) |
| Republic of Korea | DRS | 2.7 (2.1–3.4) | 14.0 (10.4–18.6) | 1400 (1000–1700) | 490 (300–700) | 1900 (1400–2300) |
| Samoa | model | 1.9 (0.0–7.5) | 13.8 (0.0–36.2) | 1 (0–2) | 0 (0–0) | 1 (0–2) |
| Singapore | DRS | 0.1 (0.0–0.6) | 2.9 (1.0–8.2) | 2 (0–9) | 1 (0–3) | 4 (0–8) |
| Solomon Islands | model | 1.9 (0.0–7.5) | 13.8 (0.0–36.2) | 18 (1–43) | 3 (0–7) | 20 (0–42) |
| Tonga | model | 1.9 (0.0–7.5) | 13.8 (0.0–36.2) | 1 (0–2) | 0 (0–0) | 1 (0–2) |
| Tuvalu | model | 1.9 (0.0–7.5) | 13.8 (0.0–36.2) | 0 (0–1) | 0 (0–1) | 1 (0–1) |
| Vanuatu | DRS | 0.0 (0.0–11.7) | 13.8 (0.0–36.2) | 5 (0–12) | 0 (0–1) | 5 (0–11) |
| Viet Nam | DRS | 2.7 (2.0–3.6) | 19.3 (14.5–25.2) | 5600 (3700–8100) | 280 (180–420) | 5900 (3800–8100) |

This report can also be downloaded at:
**http://stoptb.wpro.who.int/**